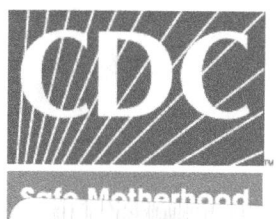

I0493900

Maternal Health Epidemiology

Reproductive Health
Epidemiology Series
Module 2

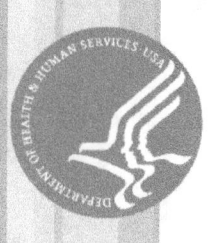

2003

DEPARTMENT OF HEALTH AND HUMAN SERVICES

MATERNAL
HEALTH
EPIDEMIOLOGY

REPRODUCTIVE HEALTH
EPIDEMIOLOGY SERIES:
MODULE 2

June 2003

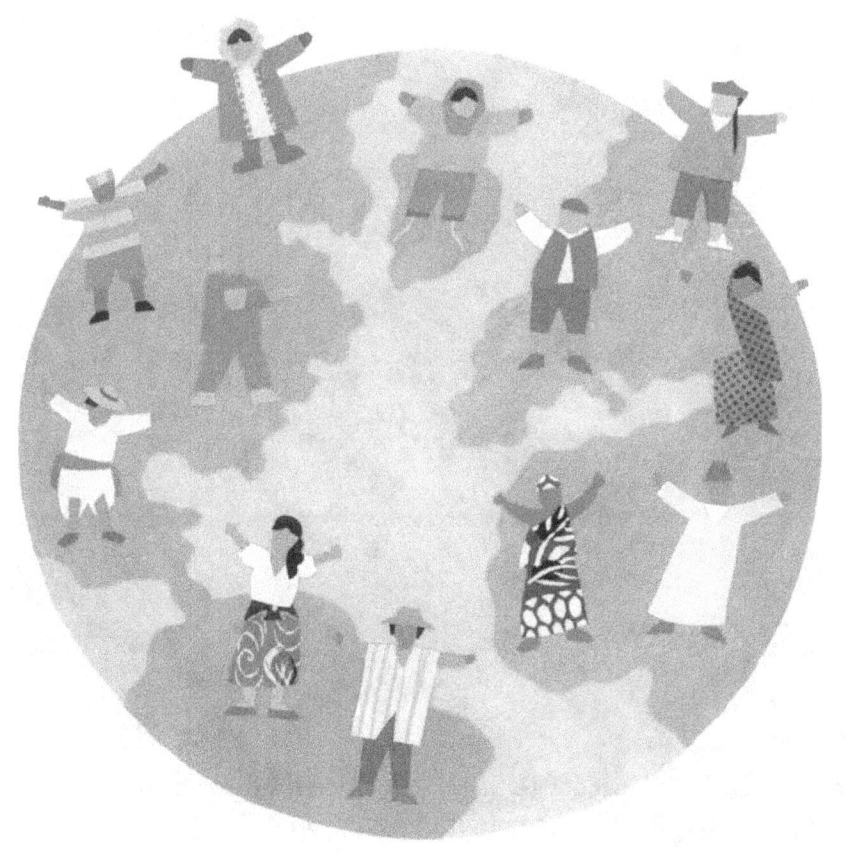

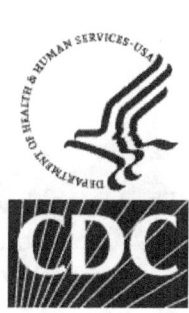

CDC

The United States Agency for International Development (USAID) provided funding for this project through a Participating Agency Service Agreement with CDC (936-3038.01).

MATERNAL HEALTH EPIDEMIOLOGY

Divya A. Patel, MPH
Nancy M. Burnett, BS
Kathryn M. Curtis, PhD

Technical Editors
Isabella Danel, MD, MS
Linda Bartlett, MD, MHSc

U.S. Department of Health and Human Services
Centers for Disease Control and Prevention
National Center for Chronic Disease Prevention and Health Promotion
Division of Reproductive Health
Atlanta, Georgia, U.S.A.
2003

CONTENTS

MATERNAL HEALTH EPIDEMIOLOGY

MATERNAL HEALTH EPIDEMIOLOGY

LEARNING OBJECTIVES

This module is designed for reproductive health professionals interested in safe motherhood (the prevention of maternal mortality and morbidity), who need a working knowledge of how epidemiology can be applied to the issue of maternal health and reducing maternal mortality and morbidity.

After studying the material in this module, the student should be able to:

- Explain how epidemiology can be applied to the issues of maternal morbidity and mortality.

- Define the main types and causes of maternal morbidity/mortality.

- List indicators used to assess maternal mortality and morbidity.

- List the steps to be taken to determine the magnitude of maternal morbidity/mortality.

- Describe sources of existing information for identifying and investigating maternal deaths.

- List the objectives of a maternal mortality surveillance system.

- List the basic steps in developing a maternal mortality surveillance system.

- Describe the elements of surveys of reproductive-age women for assessing maternal health.

- Describe the components of case-control and cohort studies for assessing maternal health.

- Discuss the major considerations in using different types of maternal health studies.

- Understand how to link indicators of maternal morbidity/mortality with program objectives.

- Describe how data on maternal health from surveillance systems, surveys, and epidemiologic studies can be linked to public health action.

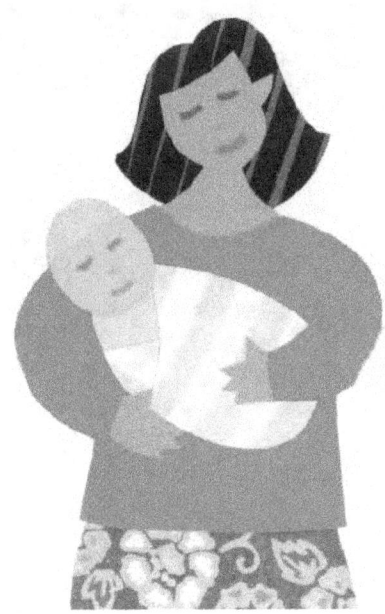

Case Study: Maternal Deaths in Abhoynagar, Bangladesh

In 1992, the number of maternal deaths in Abhoynagar, Bangladesh, was 440 per 100,000 live births. At the time, 95% of all deliveries and 80% of all maternal deaths occurred at home, most within the first 48 hours of delivery. The main causes of these maternal deaths were unsafe abortion, postpartum hemorrhage, pregnancy-induced hypertension, obstructed labor, and sepsis. To address the problem of maternal mortality, the Ministry of Health and Family Welfare (MOHFW) and the International Centre for Diarrhoeal Disease Research, Bangladesh (ICDDR, B) decided to collaborate to improve maternal health care services for women in this region.

Several interrelated interventions were initiated as part of this project. A maternity clinic that could provide basic emergency obstetric services was established, with a female physician on call 24 hours a day. Skilled community midwives were assigned to the health posts, covering a population of 20,000 each. These midwives made community antenatal visits, provided health education, detected and managed antenatal problems, organized referrals to the newly established maternity clinic, and visited new mothers as soon as possible after delivery. The government hospital, located one hour from Abhoynagar, was equipped with skilled staff, the ability to provide blood replacement, and surgical capacity to provide comprehensive emergency obstetric care. A strategy to educate traditional birth assistants to recognize complications and to know where to obtain the necessary services was outlined. To measure the effect of these interventions, a simple system of data collection was initiated by introducing a register in the maternity unit.

As a result of this combination of interrelated interventions, the number of maternal deaths dropped from 440 to 140 per 100,000 live births in the intervention area in just 3 years. The majority (80%) of the complicated cases were managed by the community midwives. In this setting, a balanced approach of upgrading services and improving women's access to these services has led to a significant decline in maternal mortality (1).

INTRODUCTION

Pregnancy and childbirth-related complications are the leading cause of disability and death among women of reproductive age in developing countries *(1)*. The death of a woman in childbirth can threaten the survival of her entire family. The development of the newborn baby who may have survived, as well as that of other young children in the family, is endangered by the death of the mother. Women who die due to pregnancy-related causes are in the prime of their lives and are responsible for the health and well-being of their families. Many women shoulder a double burden of helping to support the family by working outside the home and taking full responsibility for household duties and child care. Yet, despite this vital role played by women in society, the high level of maternal mortality in many poor countries is strong evidence of the neglect of the health needs of women.

The number of women who die each year as a result of being pregnant is not precisely known. Underreporting and misclassification of maternal deaths are universal. A large proportion of those who die are poor and live in remote, rural areas and, thus, their deaths go unreported. In regions of the world with the highest rates of maternal mortality, deaths and their causes are rarely recorded. Although hospital data indicate high rates of mortality, most of the available information is incomplete and unreliable. Moreover, relying solely on hospital or other health care facility data omits deaths that occur at home or during transport. To decide whether the death of a woman is a maternal death, the timing of the death in relation to the woman's pregnancy status, along with the cause of death, must be known *(2)*. Often, this information is not readily available. Misclassification of maternal deaths happens when the cause of death on the death certificate does not reflect the true relationship between a woman's pregnancy and her death. The combination of these factors leads to reported rates of maternal mortality that are unreliable and tend to underestimate the true magnitude of this major public health issue, making international comparisons using these data less meaningful.

Reported rates of maternal mortality underestimate the true magnitude of the problem by as much as 70% *(3)*. Even in countries where most deaths are medically certified, maternal mortality can still be significantly underestimated. For example, a study conducted in the United States by the Centers for Disease Control and Prevention (CDC) estimated that the number of deaths attributed to pregnancy and its complications from 1982 to 1996 is actually 1.3 to 3 times the rate based solely on vital statistics data *(4)*.

Underreporting and Misclassification of Maternal Mortality in Taiwan

*R*esearchers in Taiwan conducted an interview census of all registered deaths that occurred among women of reproductive age from 1984 to 1988 (5). Researchers screened pregnancy-related deaths from all collected questionnaires and death certificates. The screened pregnancy-related deaths were then reviewed by obstetrician-gynecologists, who assigned a cause of death. Results of this study revealed that, during these 5 years, the average rate of underreporting of maternal mortality was 53.4%, and, of reported deaths, only 53.3% were correctly classified with respect to cause of death.

Special efforts have to be made to obtain reliable data on maternal mortality. In the past, demographic studies focused generally on the socioeconomic determinants of maternal health, and epidemiologic surveys tended to concentrate on the biological processes of mortality and morbidity. More recently, both scientific disciplines are becoming increasingly aware of the need to integrate their work; together they may provide improved health information needed to describe the magnitude and identify the determinants of maternal mortality and morbidity, and to evaluate the impact of health interventions in a population.

To date, data on maternal mortality and morbidity have been routinely collected following a consistent methodology of collection in only certain places in the world. To make improvements in morbidity and mortality trends, baseline data need to be collected so that the impact of interventions can be more accurately assessed. These assessments help to focus the attention and resources of policymakers and decision makers by bringing to light the magnitude of women's deaths related to pregnancy. This module introduces 1) the magnitude and causes of maternal mortality and morbidity; 2) definitions of the measures of maternal mortality and morbidity; 3) methods for measuring maternal mortality; 4) epidemiologic studies to address maternal mortality and morbidity; and 5) implications of research and collected data on maternal mortality and morbidity. By studying maternal deaths, we can begin to understand what actions need to be taken at the community level, within the formal health care system, and in other social sectors to improve prevention strategies for reducing maternal morbidity and mortality.

Measures of maternal health should not focus solely on mortality. Because the factors that cause maternal deaths clearly overlap with those that cause maternal morbidity (6), interventions aimed at reducing maternal mortality will, in the process, reduce maternal morbidity as well. Useful indicators of progress toward improved maternal health status are discussed further in the section titled "Measures of Maternal Mortality and Morbidity." A few basic definitions that are useful in the discussion of maternal mortality and morbidity are provided (see Important Definitions in Maternal Mortality and Morbidity, p. 7).

Important Definitions in Maternal Mortality and Morbidity

Maternal death: *The death of a woman while pregnant or within 42 days of the termination of pregnancy, irrespective of the duration and site of pregnancy, from any cause related to or aggravated by the pregnancy or its management but not from accidental or incidental causes (ICD-10, 1993). ICD-10 also introduced two new measures of mortality temporally associated with pregnancy:*

> **Late maternal death:** *A maternal death resulting from direct or indirect obstetric causes more than 42 days but less than one year after termination of pregnancy.*

> **Pregnancy-related death:** *A maternal death occurring during pregnancy or within 42 days of termination of pregnancy, irrespective of cause.*

Maternal mortality ratio (MMR or MMRatio): *The number of maternal deaths per 100,000 live births in a given time period. The MMR expresses obstetric risk, or a woman's chances of dying from a given pregnancy. This is the most commonly used indicator of maternal health (7).*

Maternal mortality rate: *The number of maternal deaths per 1,000 women of reproductive age (usually 15–49 years). This is an indicator of the risk of maternal death among women of reproductive age and provides an indication of the burden of maternal death in the adult female population (7).*

Lifetime risk of maternal death: *The annual maternal mortality rate multiplied by the length of the reproductive period (usually 35 years). This measure reflects the cumulative risk of becoming pregnant and dying as a result of pregnancy in a woman's lifetime (7).*

Reproductive morbidity: *Illness that includes conditions of physical ill-health related to the concepts of "successful childbearing" and of "freedom from gynecological disease and risk" (8). According to this definition, reproductive morbidities can be classified as follows:*

> **Obstetric morbidity:** *Maternal illness during pregnancy, delivery, and the postpartum period.*

> **Gynecological morbidity:** *Illness of the female reproductive tract not associated with a particular pregnancy, such as reproductive tract infections, cervical cell changes, prolapse, and infertility.*

DEFINING THE PROBLEM: MAGNITUDE AND CAUSES OF MATERNAL MORTALITY AND MORBIDITY

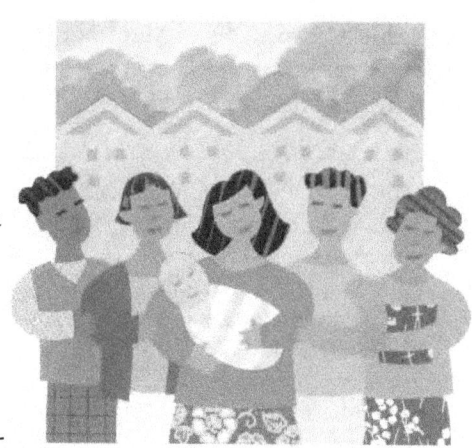

Worldwide, more than 200 million women become pregnant each year. Although most pregnancies end with a live baby to a healthy mother, in some cases, the event is a time of pain, suffering, and even death. In fact, an estimated 585,000 women die each year (Table 1), and another 20 million women develop chronic, debilitating illnesses as a result of pregnancy-related complications *(9)*. Of these maternal deaths, an estimated 99% take place in developing countries.

Throughout the world, differing behavioral and biological factors increase the risk of a woman's developing life-threatening complications. In most cultures, childbirth is surrounded by traditions, many of which are beneficial; others may be harmful to the woman and child. Maternal mortality is affected by many interrelated factors including social status and position of women, economic resources and infrastructure of the country, and the accessibility and availability of skills, materials, and facilities for appropriate family planning and obstetric care. WHO estimates that at least 15% of all pregnant women require rapid and skilled obstetric care, without which they will suffer serious, long-term morbidities *(6)*. Even so, the needs of the woman in labor sometimes go unnoticed or unrecognized. If the needed help is not available, childbirth may end in the death or permanently impaired health of the mother, infant, or both.

The major causes of maternal deaths are essentially the same around the world. The five major pregnancy-related complications leading to maternal mortality are postpartum hemorrhage, puerperal infections, hypertensive disorders of pregnancy, obstructed labor, and unsafe abortion. Table 2 summarizes WHO estimates of maternal incidence and mortality, by major obstetric complication.

Maternal Death

According to the Tenth Revision of the International Classification of Diseases (ICD-10), a maternal death is the death of a woman while pregnant or within 42 days of termination of pregnancy, irrespective of the duration and site of the pregnancy, from any cause related to or aggravated by the pregnancy or its management but not from accidental or incidental causes.

Table 1. Estimates of Maternal Mortality

United Nations region	Maternal mortality ratio*	Number of maternal deaths	Lifetime risk of maternal death, 1 in:[†]
World	430	585,000	60
More developed regions[‡]	27	4,000	1,800
Less developed regions	480	582,000	48
Africa	870	235,000	16
Eastern Africa	1,060	97,000	12
Middle Africa	950	31,000	14
Northern Africa	340	16,000	55
Southern Africa	260	3,600	75
Western Africa	1,020	87,000	12
Asia[†]	390	323,000	65
Eastern Asia	95	24,000	410
South-central Asia	560	227,000	35
South-eastern Asia	440	56,000	55
Western Asia	320	16,000	55
Europe	36	3,200	1,400
Eastern Europe	62	2,500	730
Northern Europe	11	140	4,000
Southern Europe	14	220	4,000
Western Europe	17	350	3,200
Latin America and the Caribbean	190	23,000	130
Caribbean	400	3,200	75
Central America	140	4,700	170
South America	200	15,000	140
Northern America	11	500	3,700
Oceania[‡]	680	1,400	26
Australia—New Zealand	10	40	3,600
Melanesia	810	1,400	21

*Maternal deaths per 100,000 live births.

[†]Lifetime risk (LTR) of maternal death reflects the chances of a woman dying from maternal causes over her reproductive life span, usually given as 30–35 years.

[‡]Australia, New Zealand, and Japan have been excluded from the regional totals, but are included in the total for more developed regions.

Source: World Health Organization. WHO revised 1990 estimates of maternal mortality: a new approach by WHO and UNICEF. Geneva, Switzerland: World Health Organization; 1996. p. 1–15.

Table 2. Estimated Global Incidence and Mortality From Main Obstetric Complications

Obstetric complications	Incidence (per 100 live births)	Number of cases (millions)	Number of deaths (thousands)	% of total maternal deaths
Hemorrhage	10.0	14.5	114	25.1
Sepsis	8.4	12.0	68	15.0
Hypertensive disorders of pregnancy	5.0	7.1	57	12.6
Obstructed labor	5.1	7.3	34	7.5
Unsafe abortion	13.9	19.8	61	13.4

Note: This is a global estimate and may vary in different settings. Figures may not add to total due to rounding.

Source: World Health Organization. Coverage of maternity care: a tabulation of available information. 3rd ed. Geneva, Switzerland: World Health Organization, Maternal Health and Safe Motherhood Programme, Division of Family Health; 1993.

Late Maternal Death

However, maternal deaths may also occur past this 42-day window from the time of pregnancy termination. Therefore, the ICD-10 also includes a category of late maternal death: the death of a woman from direct or indirect obstetric causes more than 42 days but less than one year after termination of pregnancy *(2)*.

Direct Maternal Death

Direct maternal deaths are deaths that result from obstetric complications of the pregnant state, which includes pregnancy, labor, and puerperium. Direct deaths can be caused by interventions, omissions, incorrect treatment, or from a chain of events resulting from a combination of these factors *(2)*. WHO estimates that the greatest proportion of maternal deaths are due to direct causes, including hemorrhage (25%), sepsis (15%), abortion (13%), hypertensive disorders of pregnancy (12%), and obstructed labor (8%) *(6)*.

Indirect Maternal Death

Indirect maternal deaths are those deaths caused by conditions or diseases that may exist before pregnancy, but are aggravated by the physiologic effects of pregnancy. About 20% of maternal deaths are due to indirect causes *(6)*. Some examples of preexisting illnesses that may be aggravated by pregnancy are heart disease, iron deficiency anemia, tuberculosis, hypertension, malaria, and diabetes mellitus.

> ### Are Maternal Deaths Due to Violence Really Coincidental?
>
> A study conducted in the USA by the Centers for Disease Control and Prevention compared injury deaths between postpartum women and other women aged 15–44 (11). Results indicated that 50% of postpartum injury deaths were homicides, compared with 26% of injury deaths among nonpregnant, nonpostpartum women. For females aged 15–19, the risk of death by homicide was 2.63 times higher for postpartum females than for other females in the same age group. There was no difference in risk of death by homicide between postpartum women and nonpregnant, nonpostpartum women when stratified separately by race and by urban/rural residence. These findings suggest an approach for prevention that includes physical abuse screening among prenatal and postpartum patients and, when necessary, referrals to services such as housing, counseling, child care, and legal assistance. Interventions that reach teenaged women in the group aged 15–19 years may be most effective in reducing postpartum injury deaths.

Pregnancy-Related Death

Incidental or "accidental" maternal deaths have historically been excluded from estimates of maternal mortality *(2)*. In practice, though, these deaths are difficult to distinguish from indirect causes of death since some of these deaths may be attributable to the pregnancy itself. For example, deaths due to homicide or suicide may be related to pregnancy for several hypothesized reasons. In places or circumstances where recording of the cause of death is unreliable, it may be useful to examine all deaths around the time of pregnancy. Therefore, the ICD-10 defines pregnancy-related death as the death of a woman while pregnant or within 43 days of termination of pregnancy, irrespective of the cause of death (2).

Puerperal Morbidity: A Neglected Area of Maternal Health in Sri Lanka

A study was conducted in three Ministry of Health areas of the Kalutara District in Sri Lanka to determine the prevalence of puerperal morbidity and to identify characteristics of those with high levels of morbidity (13). Of the mothers registered by the Public Health Midwives of the study area, 600 women were selected for the study. Data were collected using structured interviews conducted within the first week after the puerperium (43–50 days after delivery).

Results of the study revealed rates of morbidity that were much higher than expected. Excessive vaginal bleeding during the puerperium was reported by 40% of mothers, in addition to relatively minor symptoms such as breast engorgement (35%) and chills (36%) reported by many mothers. Alarmingly, only 11% of the mothers in the study did not have any symptoms or signs of illness, and the rest reported one or more symptoms. Risk factors for morbidity included first pregnancy and experiencing pregnancy wastage (pregnancy that ends in miscarriage, stillbirth, or a nonsurviving premature infant) during an earlier pregnancy.

The figures for maternal mortality alone do not tell the whole story of the suffering caused by untreated complications of pregnancy and childbirth. In some parts of the world, ill health associated with childbearing is so common that people tend to accept it as normal and virtually unavoidable, regardless of the severity. Although exact figures are not known, it is estimated that for every woman who dies, at least 30 develop chronic, debilitating problems (12). Although data on maternal mortality are more readily available than data on morbidity, it is important to keep in mind the overlap between maternal mortality and maternal morbidity—the same factors that lead to maternal deaths are responsible for the burden of maternal morbidity around the world.

A broad range of complications can occur during the puerperium, or the first 6 weeks after childbirth or abortion. Some disorders may be the result of complications that occur only during pregnancy and childbirth; others are not specific to pregnancy but may be aggravated by the pregnancy.

The debilitating sequelae of untreated pregnancy complications can be both short term and long term. Postpartum and postabortion infections, common in developing countries, can lead to pelvic inflammatory disease (PID). In addition to chronic pelvic pain and discomfort, PID can result in ectopic pregnancy, pelvic adhesions, and permanent infertility. Repeated and prolonged labors may lead to uterine prolapse, which, in turn, can cause urinary incontinence, chronic discomfort, and pain. If poorly managed, obstructed labor can cause rupturing of the uterus or obstetric fistulae, an abnormal passage between the vagina and bladder or rectum. Perhaps one of the most debilitating of morbidities, leaking urine and feces caused by obstetric fistulae, leads to painful skin rashes and a permanent odor. Along with these physical complications, women suffering from this condition may become social outcasts.

A related concept, called near miss maternal death, describes complications that become life-threatening and require immediate and adequate management to prevent. A near miss has also been described as an acute organ system dysfunction, which, if not treated properly, could result in death *(14)*. When applied to maternal health, this measure of severe acute maternal morbidity may be useful in developing interventions for conditions more likely to lead to maternal mortality. Studying near misses can be a means of identifying the major potential obstetric problems in a particular setting. Examples of life-threatening near-miss conditions are eclampsia, disseminated intravascular coagulation, and respiratory failure. Intensive care unit admission is often used as an indicator of a near-miss condition.

The advantage of using the near-miss patient is that, by definition, the woman survives and can be interviewed and observed to get a clearer picture of the events leading from good health to severe maternal morbidity. This type of study makes it possible to identify the socioeconomic and behavioral characteristics of a group of women who were very ill and required extensive medical care and resources during their treatment. If reported to clinicians, managers, and policymakers, this information could be useful in assessing the bigger picture of disease patterns among patients, planning programs, and allocating health care resources to prevent maternal deaths.

Identifying Opportunities for Preventing Maternal Deaths in South Africa

A multicenter study of academic hospitals that serve indigent women in the Pretoria Health Region was carried out to identify episodes of substandard care and missed opportunities for preventing maternal deaths (14). The study found that the most common reason for being classified as a maternal near miss was if the woman was seen at the facility for emergency gynecologic services such as abortion or ectopic pregnancy. In fact, the study found that 42 (29%) of the 147 women classified as a maternal near miss were from emergency gynecology services.

The study brought to light a major source of emergencies facing women and, hence, the area requiring the most urgent intervention in this setting. Using the near-miss definition of severe acute maternal morbidity helped researchers identify nearly five times as many cases as maternal deaths. The near-miss definition allows for an effective, easily incorporated audit system of maternal care because it is clinically based, the near-miss definition is solid, and the cases identified reflect the pattern of maternal deaths in this setting. Policymakers and health care workers in South Africa can use the information on disease patterns among their patients to design and implement appropriate interventions that will help reduce the number of near-miss maternal deaths occurring in facilities.

HOW TO DETERMINE THE MAGNITUDE OF MATERNAL MORTALITY AND MORBIDITY

Vital Records

In identifying maternal deaths, the first step is to look at existing sources of information. *Vital records* often serve as the initial source for determining the magnitude of maternal mortality in a given population. However, cause of death is routinely reported in only 78 countries or areas covering a total population of 1.8 billion, or 35% of the world's population *(15)*. Even among countries where every death is registered, maternal mortality is often still underreported due to improper recording or coding of cause of death. Identifying maternal deaths is made easier if every death is registered and each has an accurate cause of death recorded. Some countries have modified their death certificates to include a check box indicating that the woman was pregnant or had been pregnant in the previous year. Using vital records, maternal deaths can be identified from International Classification of Diseases (ICD) codes 630 to 676.9, which officially indicate pregnancy (see Appendix I for ICD codes). Even where death certificate data are computerized, a manual review of the death certificates often reveals additional cases through uncoded notes written in the margin of the certificate.

Furthermore, depending on the completeness of death registration and the accuracy of cause of death, biases may arise. Registered deaths tend to differ from those that are not registered. For example, deaths of women in urban areas or who have received better medical care are more likely to be registered than are deaths among women in rural areas or who have not received medical care *(16)*. Other pitfalls of vital registration systems include cause-of-death errors in which the cause of death listed does not specifically identify the death as maternal and delays in the collection and processing of vital records data at a national level.

Since only about one-third of the world's population lives in countries or areas where vital registration is fairly complete and the certification of cause of death is reasonably reliable *(15)*, alternative sources of information and other methods must be used to determine the magnitude of maternal morbidity and mortality where registration is incomplete or nonexistent.

Hospital Records

Generally, maternal deaths occurring in hospitals are relatively easy to identify. *Hospital records* often contain information useful in ascertaining the factors that contributed to the death. Some hospitals may have a computerized system that records admissions and deaths along with information on diagnoses that can be used as an initial screening method to capture maternal deaths. Or, if the hospital maintains a listing of deaths, a periodic review of all records of deaths among women of reproductive age would be useful in detecting maternal deaths.

One of the main problems with using hospital records is that only the deaths occurring in the hospital are identified by hospital record review. Depending on the type of hospital, the rate of maternal mortality may vary significantly. If the hospital is fee-for-service, or serves patients with a certain type of insurance, it may attract economically advantaged women. These hospitals may have a lower maternal mortality rate than that of the rest of the community. On the other hand, government (nonfee paying) hospitals may have higher maternal mortality rates because a large proportion of women who die there are admitted in emergency or high-risk conditions; in other words, they are women who had intended to give birth at home but who were transported to the hospital when their conditions became life-threatening *(3)*.

Community Identification of Deaths

Although hospital-based studies can be valuable sources of cause-of-death information, maternal deaths that occur outside the hospital are much more difficult to identify. It is important to identify and investigate deaths occurring outside the health system because these women may die of different causes than do women who die in hospitals. *Community identification of deaths* occurs when persons sometimes referred to as key informants report information from the community to the health sector *(16)*. Key informants may be traditional birth attendants, village health workers, village leaders, or simply well-connected individuals in the community.

The identification of deaths that occur in the community depends on many factors. This method requires that the informant is aware of the woman's pregnancy, the need to report the event, as well as to whom to report the event. A solid relationship between the informants and health authorities is essential, and the health system must be willing to accept the inclusion of deaths that have not been officially registered.

Formal Surveillance Systems

Formal surveillance systems are another source of information useful in detecting maternal deaths. In certain areas, the death of a woman of reproductive age or a death due to pregnancy or its complications is on the list of notifiable diseases in the government-run surveillance system. In this system, surveillance for maternal deaths is usually conducted by the epidemiology or surveillance division of the Ministry of Health instead of the local family or maternal and child health (MCH) unit. This type of surveillance system, if well-designed and functioning, can reduce many of the pitfalls associated with other methods of identifying maternal deaths. (See Methods of Measuring Maternal Mortality, p. 33.)

MEASURES OF MATERNAL MORTALITY AND MORBIDITY

Counting the number of maternal deaths is an extremely difficult task; even so, the evolution of maternal mortality research has created a need for measures of the magnitude of the problem. The universal underestimation of maternal mortality is based on two main factors: certification practices and the degree of sophistication of the vital registration system *(2)*. Although the definition of a maternal death remains constant, in practice, maternal deaths are not always captured either because the precise cause of death cannot be given or because the pregnancy may not have been noted on the death certificate.

Indicators are useful in measuring progress toward predefined health objectives, as well as evaluating the health objective itself. An indicator is a measurement that, when compared with either a standard or desired level of achievement, provides information regarding a health outcome or management process. Indicators can serve as markers of progress toward improved reproductive health status. An indicator can either be a direct measure of impact, or an indirect one, which measures progress toward specified program goals. Indicator data are collected periodically over time to track progress toward system objectives. *Impact* indicators provide information on the end result, but do not provide insight into how the outcome was achieved. For this reason, combining impact indicators with *process* (program activities) and *outcome* (results of those activities) indicators provides the best information to evaluate a surveillance system.

The issue of classification of indicators is widely debated, and definitions vary among different organizations, but process and outcome indicators are the main focus of this discussion. Process indicators are generally easier to measure than outcome measures. However, process indicators are limited in that they do not measure the effectiveness of the process, nor do they measure the event of primary interest *(15)*. Thus, process indicators may not necessarily correlate with outcome measures. Accordingly, although process indicators are useful in the short term, outcome measures ultimately must be used to measure actual changes in health status.

Across the world, the data that are collected and analyzed differ widely in terms of quality or presentation. Population-based indicators (indicators pertaining to a general population, and this population is the denominator and/or sampling frame) are the ideal measures of maternal mortality and morbidity, and of progress toward improved maternal health. In reality, the sources of data are usually

Useful Indicators in Maternal Mortality and Morbidity

Impact Indicators: Reflect changes in the primary health event of interest (i.e., morbidity, mortality), and other health outcomes.

Outcome Indicators: Reflect changes in knowledge, attitudes, behaviors, or the availability of necessary services that result from program activities.

Process Indicators: Specify the actions needed for program implementation in order to achieve the intended outcomes.

related to particular facilities or small geographic areas, which makes extrapolation to the population or national level rarely possible. Therefore, although the number of maternal deaths occurring in a particular facility or region is a useful measure of magnitude, it is difficult to interpret and generally cannot be used to make direct comparisons across time, regions, or even facilities *(3)*. Another challenge lies in determining the true numerators and denominators of outcome and process measures. For most of these measures, population-based information in both numerators and denominators would be ideal. However, since this information is typically not available, alternate estimates, or proxy measures, are often used (for example, number of live births as an estimate of the total number of pregnancies).

Impact Indicators

Although past experience has proven that measuring change in maternal mortality levels is impractical in many settings, surveillance for maternal mortality can work in some situations, but is likely to require more resources than are available in the project period to determine a significant change in the maternal mortality rate.

Impact indicators reflect changes in mortality, morbidity, and other health outcomes. A minimal list of impact indicators suggested for monitoring progress toward reducing maternal mortality is described hereafter.

Maternal Mortality

Maternal mortality ratio

Definition. The maternal mortality ratio (MMR or MMRatio) is the number of maternal deaths per 100,000 live births. The maternal mortality ratio is calculated as follows *(2)*:

$$\frac{\text{Number of maternal deaths in a given time period}}{\text{Number of live births occurring in the same time period}} \times 100{,}000$$

WHO currently recommends including maternal deaths that occur within 42 days of the end of pregnancy; countries that use other time periods are urged to use both WHO and national definitions. ICD-10 includes the category of late maternal deaths, or deaths occurring more than 42 days but less than 1 year after termination of pregnancy. The main sources of data for maternal deaths are vital registration, population-based inquiries, and health service statistics.

The numerator includes deaths due to direct obstetric complications of pregnancy, labor, or the puerperium (direct obstetric deaths) and deaths from a previously existing condition that develops during or is aggravated by the pregnancy (indirect obstetric deaths). Deaths by accidental or incidental causes, such as an automobile accident, are generally not included in the numerator. This measure of disease frequency is a ratio, not a rate, since the numerator (maternal deaths) is not a subset of the denominator (live births). The ideal measure would incorporate the total number of pregnancies (not just live births) in the denominator; however, pregnancies that result in a late fetal death or end in induced terminations are difficult to record, and data are often incomplete. As a result, the population at risk of maternal death is generally taken as the number of live births, which is assumed to be a good proxy for the number of pregnancies.

Use and Interpretation. The maternal mortality ratio, the most widely used measure of maternal mortality, measures obstetric risk once a woman becomes pregnant. It is a measure designed to indicate the likelihood that a pregnant woman will die from complications of pregnancy, childbirth, or the puerperium. The maternal mortality ratio is especially useful to measure progress in maternity services. However, because the maternal mortality ratio is not an age-standardized measure, this indicator is not completely comparable across countries.

Maternal mortality rate

Definition. The maternal mortality rate is the number of maternal deaths per 1,000 women of reproductive age. The maternal mortality rate is calculated as follows *(7)*:

$$\frac{\text{Number of maternal deaths during a given time period (generally one year)}}{\text{Number of women of reproductive age}} \times 1,000$$

The definition of reproductive age varies. WHO generally uses the age range of 15–45 years, but it is not unusual for a country to use the range of 15–49 years, or 10–45/49 where early fertility is common *(2)*. The main sources of data on maternal deaths are the same for the maternal mortality ratio: vital registration, population-based inquiries, and health service statistics.

Use and Interpretation. The maternal mortality rate measures the risk of dying and includes the likelihood of both becoming pregnant and dying during the pregnancy or the puerperium. Therefore, the maternal mortality rate measures both the risk of maternal death and the frequency with which women are exposed to this risk. This measure is useful for measuring baseline or progress in reproductive health services, since it incorporates progress in family planning use and maternity services *(19)*.

Lifetime risk of maternal death

Definition. The lifetime risk of maternal death (LTR) reflects the chances of a woman dying from maternal causes over her reproductive life span, usually given as 30–35 years. This measure is determined both by the chance of becoming pregnant (fertility) and the risk of death once pregnant (MMR). The LTR can be calculated as follows (7):

$$\frac{\text{Number of maternal deaths in 1 year}}{\text{Number of women of reproductive age}} \times 35 \text{ years}$$

In other words, the LTR is equal to the annual maternal mortality rate multiplied by 35 years of risk.

Use and Interpretation: For interpretation purposes, the reciprocal of the LTR is used more frequently than the LTR itself. For example, an LTR of 0.028 is interpreted as 1/0.028 = 36, or 1 in 36 women will die from maternal causes in her reproductive lifetime (7).

Case fatality rate

Definition. The case fatality rate (CFR) is the proportion of women with obstetric complications in a specific facility who die. The CFR is calculated as follows (17):

$$\frac{\substack{\text{Number of women with obstetric complications who die} \\ \text{in a particular facility in a given period of time}}}{\substack{\text{Number of women admitted to a facility with an obstetric} \\ \text{complication or who develop a complication while in that} \\ \text{particular facility over the same time period}}}$$

The numerator is a count of the deaths from one or more of the following complications: hemorrhage (antepartum and postpartum), prolonged or obstructed labor, postpartum sepsis, complications of abortion, preeclampsia or eclampsia, ectopic pregnancy, and ruptured uterus. The denominator is a count of cases of these complications in facilities offering essential obstetric functions (EOF) or emergency obstetric care (EmOC) during the same period. EOF at the health center level include, at minimum, provision of parenteral antibiotics, oxytocic drugs, and sedatives for eclampsia; and manual removal of placenta and retained products of conception. In addition, these services should include anesthesia, surgery, and blood transfusion at the district level. Basic EmOC includes parenteral antibiotics, oxytocic drugs, and sedatives; manual removal of the placenta; removal of retained products of conception; and assisted vaginal delivery. In addition, comprehensive EmOC includes basic EmOC, plus obstetric surgery and blood transfusions.

The complications included in both the numerator and denominator must be the same. Facility records are the main source of data for both the numerator and denominator. Maternal deaths are ascertained by the facility birth/admission/discharge register, which may also provide information on complications. The CFR is relatively easy to calculate once data on complications are being collected in the facility.

Use and Interpretation. The case fatality rate is an indicator of the likelihood that a woman with an obstetric complication will survive after admission to the medical facility. This measure will be affected by the quality and promptness of medical care provided, and the condition of the woman upon admission to the facility. In facilities where the

---

Measuring Maternal Deaths in Honduras

Studies in some countries suggest that the direct measurement of maternal deaths is feasible. With a gross national product of $740 (US) per capita, Honduras is considered one of the poorest countries in Latin America. Even so, Honduras was able to identify its maternal deaths. In 1990, the Honduran Ministry of Health conducted a study to measure mortality among women of reproductive age and found 314 maternal deaths. In 1997, a follow-up study identified 192 maternal deaths. Expected age-specific mortality rates based on life expectancy indicate that these findings correlated well with the expected number of deaths.

	1990 study	1997 study
WRA* mortality rate per 1000 WRA	1.43 (n=1757)	1.50 (n=2143)
All deaths within 42 days of pregnancy per 100,000 live births	221	150
Maternal mortality ratio (MMR)	182	115[†]
Maternal mortality rate (per 1000 WRA)	0.26	0.13

* WRA = Women of reproductive age.
[†]The reduction of the MMR from 182 to 115 is statistically significant.

The additional cost of the 1997 study was minimal, since some of the work of identifying and investigating deaths was done by departments of health as part of their routine surveillance. To supplement the work done by the departments, four female assistants were hired for 4 to 5 months each at a total cost of $8,000 (US). The assistants visited hospitals and cemeteries, met with key informants in communities, and checked vital records and forensic and autopsy logbooks to ensure that all women of reproductive age were being captured by the study. The success of the study has caused the Honduran Ministry of Health to consider incorporating this experience into its ongoing public health surveillance.

Source: Danel I. Keeping our eyes on the target—the importance of monitoring maternal mortality. MotherCare Matters 1999;8:2–3.

number of complicated cases is small, the CFR will not be stable enough to be meaningful. On the other hand, if the number of cases is large, then CFRs can be calculated for specific complications.

Although the CFR is closely related to maternal mortality at the facility level, the overall representativeness of this indicator is directly related to the proportion of women with obstetric complications who are treated in facilities. For example, it may not be useful to compare case fatality rates from a health center and a hospital, since women with the most serious complications would be referred to the hospital for last-minute, emergency care, where they would die. This tends to lower the CFR at the health center and raise the CFR at the hospital. In this way, the CFR accurately reflects the level of referrals in a particular facility. The ideal measure would be a population-based CFR, because facility-based measures are difficult to extrapolate to the general population.

Proportionate mortality

Definition. Proportionate mortality is a useful measure of the percentage of deaths among women of reproductive age that are due to pregnancy. It can be calculated as follows *(16)*:

$$\frac{\text{Number of maternal deaths during a given time period}}{\substack{\text{Number of deaths among women of reproductive age} \\ \text{during the same time period}}} \times 100$$

This measure can be further broken down to monitor particular trends in maternal mortality, referred to as cause-specific proportionate mortality.

Cause-specific proportionate maternal mortality

Definition. The cause-specific proportionate mortality can be used to compare the relative importance of a particular cause of maternal death with other causes of death. This indicator can be calculated as follows *(16)*:

$$\frac{\substack{\text{Number of maternal deaths due to a specific cause} \\ \text{in a given time period}}}{\substack{\text{Total number of maternal deaths due to all causes} \\ \text{in the same time period}}} \times 100$$

Use and Interpretation. Proportionate mortality is helpful in establishing the importance of pregnancy as a cause of death for women. Determining cause-specific proportionate maternal mortality indicators enables the monitoring of trends in causes of maternal mortality.

Example: How to Calculate the Prevalence of Third-Trimester Anemia

The prevalence of third-trimester anemia is a useful outcome measure of maternal health in many countries, since severe anemia is associated with increased risk of maternal mortality. Anemia in pregnancy is defined as a hemoglobin concentration of less than 110 g/l, and its prevalence can be calculated as follows:

$$\frac{\text{Number of women in 3rd trimester with Hb} < 110 \text{ g/dl}}{\text{Estimated number of live births}}$$

The estimated number of live births in the denominator is a proxy for the true denominator of women in the third trimester of pregnancy. Data sources for this indicator include surveillance/routine reporting and surveys. Periodic assessment of the prevalence of anemia will help to identify the best mix of strategies for reducing anemia in a population.

Adapted from: World Health Organization. Mother-baby package: implementing safe motherhood in countries. Geneva, Switzerland: World Health Organization, Maternal Health and Safe Motherhood Programme, Division of Family Health; 1996.

Both the cause-specific proportionate maternal mortality and the proportionate mortality work best when data on cause of death are relatively accurate, and identification and classification of deaths remain consistent. A drawback of these measures is that they do not provide information on changes in risk. For example, the maternal mortality due to a particular cause may decrease while the overall proportionate mortality stays the same.

Maternal Morbidity

Prevalence and incidence of maternal complications and sequelae

Definition. The measures of disease most often used in epidemiology are prevalence and incidence. The point prevalence of a maternal complication is the proportion of women of reproductive age who have the complication, and can be calculated as follows:

$$\frac{\text{Number of existing cases of particular maternal complication at a specified point in time}}{\text{Population at risk}} \times 100$$

All women who have the complication at the specified time are included in the numerator, regardless of the length of time they had the complication. The denominator includes the total population at risk—for example, all pregnant women under study. The total population can be estimated by the number of live births in a time period as a surrogate measure of all pregnancies.

The incidence of maternal complications, by contrast, is the number of new cases of the complication that occur in the population at risk within a specified period of time. The incidence rate can be calculated as follows:

$$\frac{\text{Number of new cases of particular maternal complication at a specified point in time}}{\text{Population at risk}} \times 100$$

Outcome and Process Indicators

Considering the limitations in measurement of impact indicators, researchers and policymakers have begun using outcome and process indicators to measure progress in reducing maternal mortality. Since both the maternal mortality ratio (MMR) and the severity of maternal morbidity can be difficult to measure, WHO, UNFPA, and UNICEF have developed outcome and process indicators to measure change in program outcomes (17). These indicators are used to measure access to and use of care, as well as quality of care (17). Outcome and process indicators are generally easier to measure than impact indicators. However, outcome and process indicators are limited in that they do not measure the event of primary importance: maternal mortality (18). It is important to remember that these indicators do not necessarily correlate with impact measures. So, although outcome and process indicators are useful in the short term, concerted efforts must still be made to improve measurements of maternal mortality using impact indicators.

What follows is a minimal list of maternal health outcome and process indicators.

Who delivers the woman, and where does the birth take place?

Definition. The first part of the measure is defined as the proportion of deliveries attended by skilled personnel. Skilled birth attendants include physicians, nurses, midwives, and trained primary health care and other workers. It can be calculated as follows (17):

$$\frac{\text{Deliveries by skilled health personnel irrespective of outcome}}{\text{All live births during the same time period and in the same geographic area as numerator}} \times 100$$

The second part of the measure is defined as the proportion of births by site (e.g., home, health center, or hospital), and can be calculated as follows *(17)*:

$$\frac{\text{Deliveries by site}}{\substack{\text{All live births during the same time period and} \\ \text{in the same geographic area as numerator}}} \times 100$$

A common source of data for this set of measures is a population-based survey, such as the Demographic and Health Survey (DHS), since these typically include only women with live births. In countries where public facilities provide most of the care, such data may be ascertained from the routine health information system of the Ministry of Health.

Use and Interpretation. This set of measures is relatively easy to collect and, when used together, can determine the progression from home births with traditional attendants, to home births with skilled attendants, to facility birthing with skilled attendants in a particular geographic area. Unfortunately, these two indicators are rarely combined to show such progression *(17)*.

The *skilled health personnel* indicator has been used extensively at global and national levels to depict the progression of birth attendants over time. For example, WHO considers the measurement of births with skilled attendants over time to be an important indicator among developing countries. The DHS has shown the increase in use of skilled attendants in several countries, using country data collected in two time periods. Distinguishing between births at home, health centers, and hospitals can provide useful data for understanding accessibility and coverage of care. Noting the split between public and private facilities also provides useful information for planning intervention strategies.

Cesarean section rate

Definition. The cesarean section rate is defined as the proportion of women who have a cesarean section in a specific geographic area in a given period of time. This indicator can be calculated as follows *(17)*:

$$\frac{\substack{\text{Number of pregnant women with cesarean section} \\ \text{during a specific time period and in} \\ \text{the same geographic area}}}{\substack{\text{Number of live births during the same time period} \\ \text{and in the same geographic area as numerator}}} \times 100$$

The numerator can be determined from birth registers in all facilities in a given geographic area. Some sources have suggested the use of a maximum rate of 15% for the percentage of deliveries by cesarean section—rates less than 5% may indicate inadequate availability or access to obstetric care or both, and rates above 15% may suggest overutilization for nonessential reasons *(19)*. The numerator can also be estimated through population-based surveys, using only the last pregnancy. The denominator is an estimate of live births that is obtained by multiplying the population by the crude birth rate. A denominator using all births (i.e., not just the last pregnancy) in a given time period would provide a population-based measure; however, this number is difficult to determine.

Collecting the information from facility registers may be more practical for yearly levels. To ensure population-based rates, registers from all facilities providing cesarean sections in the geographic area must be included (both public and private providers). On the other hand, the use of population-based surveys has the advantage that fewer cesarean section cases may be missed. The validity of self-reported cesarean sections is questionable because some women have reportedly mistaken episiotomies for cesarean sections, causing the cesarean section rate to be overestimated *(17)*.

Use and Interpretation. The cesarean section rate is considered a useful indicator of availability and access to emergency services, as well as the functioning of the health service system. The rate, or access to cesarean section, is considered a necessary component of quality of maternal care. Access to cesarean section capabilities can be revealed through comparing rates of urban and rural populations. Compared with other maternal health process indicators, cesarean section data are relatively reliable; however, the appropriateness of cesarean sections is difficult to determine since most registers do not indicate why a cesarean section was performed.

Met need for essential obstetric services

Definition. Met need for essential obstetric services (EOC) is defined as the proportion of cases of major obstetric complications that are appropriately managed in a specific geographic area in a given period of time *(17)*. EOC includes the means to manage emergency complications as well as procedures for early detection and treatment to prevent problem pregnancies from progressing to emergencies. It can be calculated as follows *(17)*:

$$\frac{\text{Number of appropriately managed cases of major obstetric complications during a specific time period and geographic area}}{\text{Number of cases of major obstetric complications estimated for the same time period and geographic area}} \times 100$$

Uses of the Met Need Indicator in Countries

The met need indicator has been used for supervision at the municipality level in Bolivia and at the district hospital level in Guatemala. It has been used for advocacy at the district level in Indonesia and Guatemala, and at the national level in Cambodia and Morocco (17).

In practice, admissions of, or consultations with, a woman with major obstetric complications is a more accurate description of the numerator, rather than the number of women with obstetric complications, because the same woman may have two or more admissions to a facility. Experts convened by WHO estimated that 15% of women with live births may suffer a major obstetric complication *(17)*. However, this method of estimation assumes that direct obstetric complications are constant across countries. The denominator, the number of women with major direct obstetric complications, can be calculated by multiplying the crude birth rate (CBR) for the country by the population of the geographic area of interest. Women living in the same geographic area should be included in both the numerator and denominator of this indicator, since past experience shows that referral hospitals may draw their patients from a wide area and thus inflate the numerator. The calculation of the numerator requires an address for each woman in the birth registry and the exclusion of women residing outside the study areas.

The broad definition of major complications includes direct obstetric complications (hemorrhage, dystocia, hypertensive disorders of pregnancy, and sepsis) and may include women with severe anemia and multiple gestation. The researcher should specify whether or not postabortion complications are included, since postabortion complications vary over time and by site.

Use and Interpretation. Met need measures the frequency with which services for any direct maternal complication are used in a specific geographic area and period of time. By holding the definitions of both the numerator and denominator constant (e.g., a specific list of direct obstetric complications in the numerator and 15% of live births in the denominator), patterns of access and use of services across districts can be examined as a measure of progress in use of services over time. It is only possible to use the met need indicator to compare countries if the same definitions (numerator and denominator) are used among the countries and if the definitions are similarly interpreted by the providers recording the data.

Referral rate

Definition. The referral rate is the proportion of women with potential or actual obstetric complications moving from one level of care to another *(17)*. It can be calculated as follows *(17)*:

$$\frac{\text{Number of women with a potential or actual obstetric complication moved to another site for care within a given time frame and geographic area}}{\text{Number of all women with obstetric complications (or deliveries or live births) within the same time period and geographic area as in the numerator}} \times 100$$

The referral rate could focus on either women referred from a site, or women received at a site due to referral. Due to the variations in types of referrals, this indicator can be either population-based (data gathered through surveys) or facility-based (data gathered from registers). The following are possible referrals:

1. Self/family referral to

  • Traditional birth attendant/community health worker.
  • First-level skilled health care provider.
  • Basic EOC facility.
  • Comprehensive EOC facility.

2. Traditional birth attendant/community health worker referral to

  • First-level skilled delivery care provider.
  • Basic EOC facility.
  • Comprehensive EOC facility.

3. First-level skilled delivery care (SDC) referral to

  • Basic EOC facility.
  • Comprehensive EOC facility.

4. Comprehensive EOC facility referral to

  • Tertiary center.

The focus of the numerator is on women with actual complications since it is not known how to estimate the number of women with potential complications. Because the use of risk factors, such as women with previous poor pregnancy outcome, has not proved to be of predictive value, only those women with complications diagnosed by a provider are currently counted. In terms of the denominator, community-level data should include all live births, whereas a facility-based referral rate would include all deliveries in the facility or all women with complications diagnosed in the facility. Sources of data on referrals in the community or at a specific facility include health facility registers, antenatal cards, delivery records, vehicle log books, special referral forms, community surveys, and community data collection systems.

Use and Interpretation. Referral rates measure access to and quality of care in a particular facility. The most useful information has come from facility-level registers for a single complication or a defined group of conditions, expressed as a percentage of deliveries or of women with complications in the facility. Referral rates are not useful for comparisons across facilities, districts, or countries.

Increased referral rates are interpreted as positive if they indicate an increased recognition of life-threatening conditions, improved decision making at the community and EOC levels, or a previous low level of utilization. Increased rates are seen as negative if they indicate that the Basic EOC level has been bypassed for reasons such as the loss of key personnel, diminishing resources, or use of inappropriate criteria for referral.

Decreased referral rates are interpreted as positive if they signify increased skills at the Basic level or a previous overload at the Comprehensive level. However, decreased rates are interpreted as negative if they correspond to a loss of confidence in the Comprehensive level, a deterioration in the system of transportation, or unaffordable health care costs.

METHODS OF MEASURING MATERNAL MORTALITY

How Do We Collect the Information Necessary for Calculating Maternal Mortality Indicators?

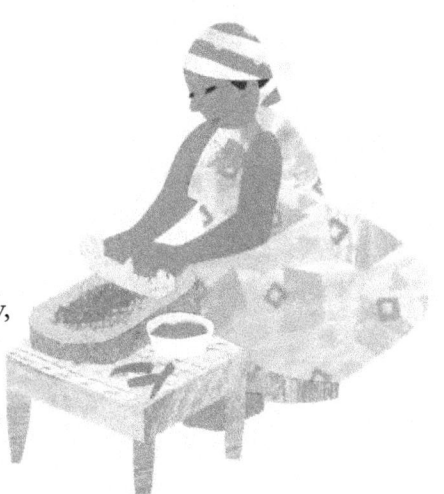

Indicators of maternal mortality described above can be challenging to calculate even when civil registration is reasonably reliable. Ideally, every maternal death would be captured and investigated. However, sentinel case methodology makes it possible to understand the magnitude and causes of the problem in a way that will enhance the development and evaluation of interventions. The identification of maternal deaths involves the following steps:

A. Conduct sentinel case surveillance for maternal deaths.

B. Conduct facility-based surveillance for maternal deaths.

C. Identify all deaths occurring among women of reproductive age (generally considered to be women aged 15–44) in the population.

   1. Establish which deaths occurred among women during or within 42 days after pregnancy.

   2. Investigate all deaths among women during or within 42 days of pregnancy.

   3. Determine which deaths were caused by pregnancy or childbirth and its complications or management.

This process is simplified in areas with complete and reliable civil registration systems. However, since nearly two thirds of the world's population lives in areas where the registration of births and deaths is incomplete or nonexistent, alternative methods are needed to obtain the relevant information for calculating indicators of maternal health. Relying on vital statistics alone leads to an underestimation of maternal mortality. Instead, multiple sources of data are needed to identify and obtain the greatest amount of information on every maternal death. A variety of methods, each with its own advantages and limitations, are described below:

A. Maternal mortality surveillance.

B. Reproductive age mortality surveys (RAMOS).

C. Surveys of reproductive-age women and household surveys.

D. Other methods.

   1. The sisterhood method.

   2. Verbal autopsy.

   3. Qualitative research.

E. Epidemiologic studies, including:

1. Cohort studies.

2. Case-control studies.

Maternal Mortality Surveillance

In some countries, maternal mortality is on the list of notifiable diseases that must be reported to the government-run surveillance system in a timely manner. To assess the magnitude of the problem, a surveillance system that captures regularly reported maternal deaths can be established. Maternal mortality epidemiologic surveillance (MMES) has been defined as "a component of the health information system, which permits the identification, notification, quantification, and determination of the causes and avoidability of maternal deaths, for a defined time period and geographic location, with the goal of orienting the measures necessary for its prevention" *(16)*.

Basic Steps in Maternal Mortality Surveillance

Death of a woman of reproductive age

↓

Identification of case as a maternal death

↓

Investigation of medical and nonmedical causes of death and determination of avoidability

↓

Analysis of data

↓

Actions: dissemination of recommendations, interventions, and evaluation

Source: Berg et al. Guidelines for maternal mortality epidemiological surveillance. Washington: The World Bank; 1996.

The primary goal of MMES is to obtain information to guide public health efforts in reducing maternal mortality. MMES involves identifying and, subsequently, investigating all deaths caused by pregnancy, its complications and management. The following are specific objectives of MMES:

• Collect accurate data on all maternal deaths.

• Analyze the data for trends in maternal mortality, causes of death, avoidability of deaths, and risk factors.

• Make informed recommendations for actions to decrease maternal mortality.

• Disseminate the findings and recommendations to policymakers, health providers, and the community.

- Evaluate the impact of interventions.

- Increase awareness about the magnitude, social effects, and preventability of maternal mortality.

- Assure that maternal mortality statistics at regional, national, and international levels are comparable.

- Identify key areas in need of further research and help establish priorities for that research.

An accurate assessment of the magnitude of the problem will enhance the ability of policymakers and decision makers to focus their attention and resources on the issue of maternal mortality. Sources of information for MMES include death certificates, hospital records, community identification of deaths, and formal surveillance systems.

What Is the Current Scope of Surveillance, and What Can Be Done to Expand It?

Finding all deaths of women of reproductive age and determining the relationship to pregnancy and childbirth is a necessary step in finding all maternal deaths. A relatively simple modification to an existing vital registration system is to include a pregnancy check box on the death certificate. This box can be checked if the woman was pregnant or had been pregnant in the previous year. All death certificates with this box checked can then be followed up to determine whether this was in fact a maternal death *(16)*.

However, some countries do not have the ability or resources required to carry out national surveillance for maternal mortality. In these situations, sentinel cases can be identified and investigated as a first step in the development of a surveillance system. In addition, maternal deaths occurring in hospitals are commonly used for estimating maternal mortality.

The surveillance of all maternal deaths could then be initiated in a pilot area, such as a region of particularly high maternal mortality or an area in which interventions can be easily implemented. However, hospital rates may not be representative of the rates in the overall population because many maternal deaths occur outside the hospital. Hospital data may include a higher proportion of high-risk women, in other words, women who intended to deliver at home but are transported to the hospital for emergency obstetric care. Fee-for-service facilities may attract economically advantaged women, thus leading to a lower maternal mortality rate than that of the overall population.

Investigating Maternal Mortality in Brazzaville, Congo

Law in Brazzaville, Congo, requires the delivery of all bodies to a mortuary before burial (21), which provides an ideal system for investigating maternal deaths. In this study, researchers investigated all bodies handled by the city's three mortuaries and interviewed relatives who delivered the bodies. For those bodies of women previously admitted to a hospital, the researchers assessed hospital files and interviewed medical staff shortly after death. Using the WHO definition of a maternal death, 15 maternal deaths were identified among the 138 female bodies aged 15–49.

Using the number of live births and the age distribution of mothers, researchers were able to directly estimate the rate of maternal mortality to be 645 per 100,000 and the lifetime risk of maternal death to be 1 in 25 women. Surveillance for maternal deaths in Brazzaville, Congo, revealed an exceptionally high maternal mortality rate for an African capital in which about 90% of the women have access to prenatal care, and most babies are delivered in maternity hospitals. It was found that the excess mortality was largely due to the high number of abortion-related deaths in young women, which were freely disclosed during interviews with family members at the mortuary.

Some countries have begun to include late maternal deaths, i.e., deaths up to 1 year after delivery, in their expanded maternal mortality surveillance systems. Another possibility that is currently being pilot tested is a system designed to identify all pregnant women who register for antenatal care and prospectively monitor their pregnancies. Certain countries with very few maternal deaths are examining ways to identify near misses, in other words, pregnant or postpartum women with severe morbidities that could have led to death. Other countries are expanding their surveillance to assess the impact of pregnancy on nonmaternal causes of death such as suicide, homicide, unintentional injuries, and HIV infection.

What Are Some Issues in Sustaining Maternal Mortality Surveillance?

Many countries have surveillance mechanisms in place for reportable illnesses or deaths, particularly polio and measles. In some countries, key informants provide information on these cases. The MMES infrastructure is most likely to be sustainable and acceptable if it is incorporated with an existing surveillance system that has proven successful.

In this example (see Investigating Maternal Mortality in Brazzaville, Congo, p. 36), investigation of maternal deaths was integrated with the existing system of surveillance, providing an effective means of determining the cause of excess maternal mortality in this setting.

It is important that the local health staff not be overwhelmed with too much work. If the caseload is unmanageable, an option is to investigate a random sample of maternal deaths. Tasks should be realistic and feasible given the available resources. On the other hand, if few maternal deaths are occurring at the local level, attention and resources may be diverted to other problems that are less serious but more common. An important aspect of sustaining MMES activity is the knowledge that efforts at the local level will have an impact at regional and national levels. Further, participation in surveillance activities is more likely to continue if action is taken on concerns raised at the local level.

An important issue in maternal mortality surveillance is the high turnover of health personnel. Since local health units are often staffed by physicians and nurses fulfilling short-term social service requirements, new staff must be trained in MMES each year. This gap in continuity of surveillance staff may lead to decreased rates of reported maternal deaths or may interfere with the ability to sustain MMES.

If reducing maternal mortality is considered a priority, resources must be allocated to operate an effective surveillance system to capture maternal deaths. The most expensive components of MMES are personnel training and the investigation of cases; however, if MMES can be integrated into other ongoing surveillance systems, the additional cost may be minimized. (For more detail on designing and implementing reproductive health surveillance systems, see *Public Health Surveillance Applied to Reproductive Health* Module.)

Reproductive Age Mortality Surveys (RAMOS)

A reproductive age mortality survey (RAMOS) identifies and investigates

---

Maternal Mortality Among Afghan Refugees in Pakistan, 1999–2000: An Application of the Reproductive Age Mortality Survey (RAMOS)

As refugee populations continue to grow around the world, information about their health status is needed to plan and evaluate health interventions. A reproductive age mortality survey (RAMOS) was undertaken among Afghan refugees living in Pakistan to determine the burden of deaths among women due to maternal causes, risk factors for deaths among women of reproductive age, whether these deaths were preventable, and barriers to health care. Data were collected in two phases. From May through September 2000, a survey of 16,247 refugee families was conducted. Information recorded through this survey included any deaths that occurred between January 1999 and August 2000, and the age and gender of the persons who had died. During the second phase of data collection, all deaths among women of reproductive age identified in the survey were investigated through verbal autopsies. Investigators interviewed surviving family members to collect information about cause of death, potential risk factors for death, preventability, and barriers to health care access. Any available medical records and medicines were also examined. The data were then reviewed to determine cause of death, whether the death was pregnancy-related, and if so, whether it was a direct or indirect maternal death.

Among 134,406 Afghan refugees, 1,197 deaths were identified, for a crude mortality rate of 5.5 (95% CI, 5.2–5.8) per thousand. Of these deaths, 66 were of women of reproductive age, and 27 were determined to be maternal deaths. The maternal mortality ratio was 291 per 100,000 live births, with a lifetime risk of maternal death of 1 in 50. Maternal causes were the single largest cause of death—41% of all deaths of women of reproductive age. Hemorrhage was the most frequent cause of direct maternal death. Of the maternal deaths, 67% were determined to be preventable, and for 81%, at least one barrier to health care was reported. From these results, recommendations were made for this specific population of Afghan refugees (e.g., preventing and treating anemia and malaria among pregnant women) and for refugee populations and humanitarian efforts worldwide (e.g., improving the availability of comprehensive emergency obstetric care services and designating a vehicle for emergency access to health care).

Source: Bartlett LA, Jamieson DJ, Kahn T, Sultana M, Wilson HG, Duerr A. Maternal mortality among Afghan refugees in Pakistan, 1999–2000. Lancet 2002;359:643–49.

Using a National Survey to Detect the Impact
of Policy Changes in Romania

National surveys provide a means to study the impact of policy changes on maternal health by comparing aspects of fertility, abortion, and contraceptive use before and after the institution of the policy. In Romania, a law issued in 1966 reversed the legal status of abortion and restricted the use of modern contraception and induced abortion to limited medical and social reasons (22). To get a clearer picture of the impact of the abortion legislation on maternal health, researchers conducted the national Romania Reproductive

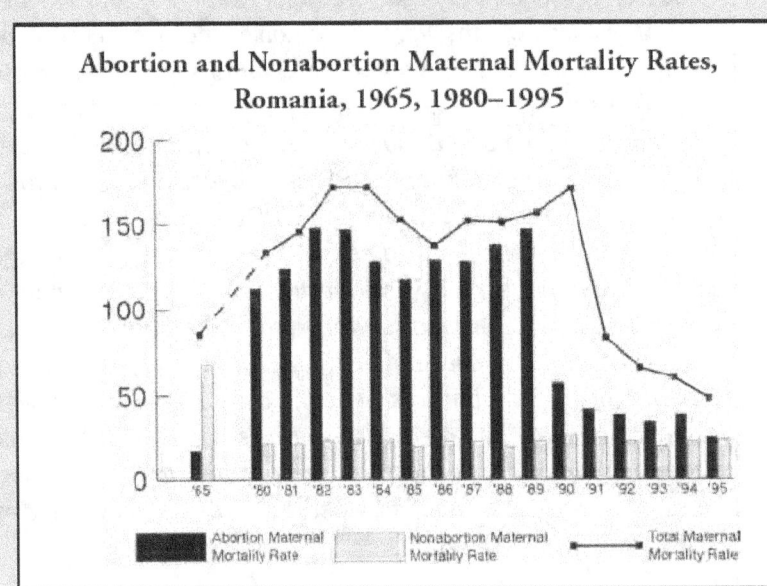

Abortion and Nonabortion Maternal Mortality Rates, Romania, 1965, 1980–1995

Health Survey (RRHS) in 1993, the first nationwide probability survey to be carried out in Romania since 1978. The survey collected information from women of reproductive age on a wide range of topics related to knowledge and attitudes surrounding reproductive health, including a history of all pregnancies and births, family planning use, maternal and child health status, uses of women's health services, knowledge of AIDS transmission and prevention, and socioeconomic characteristics of the women and their husbands and families. Information from the RRHS pregnancy histories was used to examine two consecutive 3-year periods before and after the restriction of abortion was repealed in 1989.

Before the 1966 law went into effect, Romanian women had access to safe abortion provided by the country's health care system, and the MMR was similar to those of other Eastern European countries (23). After the legislation, the MMR in Romania rose sharply to a level 10 times that of any other European country and remained high for several years, with more than 85% of the deaths related to abortion (see graph).

In December 1989, during the Romanian revolution, the restrictive law banning abortion and contraception was repealed due to public pressure on the interim government. The effect of switching from unsafe, illegal abortions back to legal abortions is dramatically reflected in the decline of the MMR: from 170 per 100,000 live births in 1989 to 60 per 100,000 live births in 1992 (see graph). This decrease was almost entirely due to the sharp decline in abortion-related deaths (21). The RRHS proved to be a useful method of examining the extent to which abortion legislation affected the health of women in Romania.

all deaths of women of reproductive age to determine the extent and causes of maternal mortality *(2)*. RAMOS is based on the general principle that no single source identified all deaths, and therefore, multiple sources of death are examined. Data collection occurs in two phases. In the first phase, all deaths of women of reproductive age are identified through review of the total deaths in the community. Sources of deaths vary from country to country, but include civil registers, hospitals and health centers, census data where families are asked about any deaths within a specific time period, village health workers, community leaders, religious authorities, and cemetery records. While one source of data may be sufficient to identify all deaths, RAMOS generally relies on several sources. Once all deaths of women of reproductive age are identified, the second phase of data collection and review begins. Investigators collect as much information as possible about the causes and circumstances of each death through a variety of techniques. Death certificates and medical records are reviewed when available. Verbal autopsies are frequently conducted to gather information from the woman's relatives, friends, and health workers (see page 42 for more information on verbal autopsies). After this information is gathered, a specialized panel determines the cause of each death and whether or not the death was pregnancy-related.

RAMOS can provide results that estimate the magnitude of maternal mortality and other causes of death of women of reproductive age, assess the burden of maternal causes of death relative to other causes, and provide information to assess the need to improve the quality of health care service to prevent maternal deaths. RAMOS has been called the "gold standard" for estimating maternal mortality *(2)*. However, this is only true in cases where every effort is made to identify all deaths in the community.

More information about RAMOS can be found in the MEASURE Evaluation Compendium of Maternal and Newborn Health Tools (www.cpc.unc.edu/measure/cmnht/cmnht.html).

Surveys of Reproductive-Age Women and Household Surveys

Reproductive health surveys can be useful sources of information regarding maternal mortality and morbidity. Information that can be ascertained from surveys includes disease status, behaviors associated with disease, risk factors, and health services data. Reproductive health surveys can be either one-time, cross sectional surveys, or large-scale, periodic surveys. These types of surveys are routinely conducted by developed countries; however, the expense of conducting such surveys is a serious limitation for developing countries. At the request of international donors, the Division of Reproductive Health (DRH) at the U.S. Centers for Disease Control and Prevention (CDC) is providing technical assistance for developing countries to implement these surveys. The Demographic and Health Surveys (DHS) program, designed to collect data on fertility, family planning, and maternal and child health, is a similar program implemented by Macro International, Inc., in several developing countries.

Although surveys can provide high-quality data, they can be time-consuming and expensive to conduct, especially on a regular basis. The information obtained from household surveys is usually not current but instead provides a maternal mortality ratio for some time in the past. Another problem with this approach is the large number of households that have to be contacted to derive reliable estimates of maternal mortality. Even when large sample sizes are used, a very small number of maternal deaths are identified. Even in high mortality settings, maternal deaths are relatively rare events *(2)*.

One-time surveys do not provide information that can be used for assessing trends. For the purposes of maternal mortality surveillance, ongoing surveys are more useful because rates can be monitored over time in a specific region. However, the data obtained is not always relevant for calculating direct estimates of maternal mortality, so reproductive health surveys should be considered a rough tool for estimating maternal mortality. Despite the limitations, in areas without formal surveillance systems for maternal mortality and morbidity, surveys provide the only method of obtaining population-based information on non-notifiable diseases—for example, information on women who do not seek care at a health facility can still be captured by a population-based survey. The best measures are ascertained from surveys conducted in regions of high fertility and high maternal mortality. The usefulness of household and reproductive health surveys can be further enhanced by the addition of certain questions or sources of data, as in the sisterhood method and verbal autopsy method, discussed in the next section.

Sisterhood Method

In some settings, estimates of maternal mortality cannot be obtained through direct methods of measurement. The sisterhood method is an indirect method that derives a variety of maternal mortality indicators from asking adults during a census or survey about their adult sisters who died during pregnancy, childbirth, or the puerperium. This method makes use of information obtained by the addition of questions on maternal deaths to demographic or community-based household surveys *(2)* to estimate a lifetime risk of maternal mortality.

Using this method, a representative sample of adults are asked questions regarding the survivorship of their sisters. The MMR can be estimated using some additional information on fertility. The following questions are added to household surveys and, along with the 5-year age group of the respondent, provide the basic information for the calculation of lifetime chances of death from maternal causes:

- The number of sisters (born to the same mother) who have reached the age of 15 years and were ever married (or, in some situations, cohabitating).

- The number of those sisters who are still alive.

- The number of sisters who have died.

- The number of deceased sisters who died while they were pregnant, during childbirth, or within 6 weeks of termination of pregnancy.

The sisterhood method is useful in areas where the alternative data sources and approaches to estimation are inadequate, for example, in areas where maternal deaths are poorly registered in official statistics. One of the main advantages of using this method is that it minimizes the number of households that must be visited to obtain information on a large number of women. The method is relatively easy to use in the field and requires smaller sample sizes than traditional direct methods.

One of the main problems with the sisterhood method is that it yields no information on the causes or circumstances surrounding the maternal deaths *(15)*. Moreover, this method can give only a retrospective

How Reliable Is the Sisterhood Method for Estimating Maternal Mortality?

*A*dults visiting any one of 91 health centers or posts in a rural region of Nicaragua were randomly sampled, and 9,232 adults were interviewed by health personnel *(24)*. So the results could be compared, the basic sisterhood method questions used were identical to those in a previous household study: 1) How many sisters have you ever had who were born to your mother and who reached the age of 15 years? 2) How many of these sisters who reached the age of 15 are still living? 3) How many of these sisters who reached the age of 15 have died? 4) How many of these dead sisters died while pregnant, in childbirth, or in the 6 weeks after a pregnancy ended? Based on the data collected using the sisterhood method, the lifetime risk of maternal death was 0.0144, or 1 in 69, and the maternal mortality ratio was 241 per 100,000 live births.

Characteristics of health facility users were not different from those of the overall population, thus allowing for the results to be generalized to other settings. The sisterhood method figures were essentially identical to the estimates of lifetime risk of maternal death of 0.0145 and the maternal mortality ratio of 243 per 100,000 obtained from the household-based survey in the same region just 8 months earlier. Comparison of the results of the two methods shows that the sisterhood method provided a good estimate of the magnitude of maternal mortality in this setting. Based on the results of this study, the use of opportunistic settings should be considered as a low-cost and efficient alternative to larger-scale, demographic surveys for estimating maternal mortality.

The Use of Verbal Autopsy to Assess Maternal Mortality in Guinea-Bissau

*D*ecision makers must have access to reliable data on the magnitude and causes of maternal mortality so that limited resources can be allocated to the most effective programs (25). Because a large proportion of the births and birth-related deaths in Guinea-Bissau occur without the involvement of a medically trained health care worker, researchers decided to collect information using verbal autopsy, a form of postmortem interview. Their aim was to develop a postmortem interview technique that would enable a local nurse with basic training to classify deaths of women of reproductive age.

To get reliable data, 100 clusters of 100 women of reproductive age (a total sample of 10,000 women) were randomly selected. The researchers developed a structured interview with filter questions, which was applied to all deaths of women of reproductive age and followed over a period of 6 years. The cause of death was ascertained by a series of diagnostic algorithms for the most common causes of maternal mortality, including postpartum and antepartum hemorrhage, puerperal infection, obstructed labor, eclampsia, abortion, and ectopic pregnancy. During this period, 350 deaths to women of reproductive age were reported, of which 32% were maternal. Using the diagnostic algorithm, 70% of the maternal deaths could be given a specific diagnosis.

The researchers were also interested in identifying the factors that are critical for obtaining sufficient information to reach a diagnosis; in other words, factors that would decrease the percentage of maternal deaths that were left unclassified. It was found that the most useful information was obtained from respondents who were present during the last illness, if the respondent was the husband of the deceased woman, and if the death occurred within 1 week after delivery. In contrast to methods by which a panel of medical experts establish the cause of death, the researchers concluded that the verbal autopsy is an economically and technically viable option in areas where health care workers have minimal training.

estimate for the MMR for the past 10–12 years (20). Although the sisterhood method can be used to set a baseline, it cannot provide an estimate for change at the end of a short period because the estimate is a weighted average of mortality conditions over a lengthy period of time (2). Further, the sisterhood method relies on the idea that siblings maintain contact throughout their lives. This assumption may not be true in settings where women leave the maternal home upon marriage and perhaps migrate to other parts of the country. The sisterhood method tends to underreport early pregnancy deaths, especially those related to abortion or those that occur among unmarried women. Such sensitive issues will always be difficult to address and, hence, underreporting pervades all methods for measuring maternal mortality.

Verbal Autopsy

Since many deaths occur without previous contact with the health system, conventional analyses using death certificates may not give accurate estimates of maternal mortality. In these areas, it may be more feasible to ascertain information on maternal deaths using a form of postmortem interview called verbal autopsy. The verbal autopsy method uses information about symptoms and signs observed before death by relatives or associates of deceased women to determine the causes of maternal deaths (25). Investigators attempt to find the closest relative and the birth attendant if the death was associated with a delivery. A structured interview is then administered that addresses issues such as place of death, care-seeking behavior, and respondent's relation to the deceased. If the death occurred within 42 days of termination of pregnancy, the interviewer uses particular responses to guide further questions regarding signs and symptoms preceding the woman's death. The final diagnosis is then derived using predefined diagnostic algorithms based on the duration, severity, and sequence of symptoms.

Verbal autopsies can be done in institutions (called case reviews) or in the community. This method allows more data to be collected to determine why a woman died. The verbal autopsy approach addresses the role of delays in identifying the problem, the decision to seek care, and whether the availability of transportation to the facility contributed to the maternal death *(26)*.

In certain settings maternal deaths are unlikely to be evaluated by a gynecological or obstetric specialist, the verbal autopsy method enables a local nurse or other health care worker with basic training to categorize deaths among women of reproductive age. However, diagnoses from the verbal autopsy method are prone to inaccuracies because they rely on the ability of respondents to observe, remember, and report the circumstances, symptoms, and signs that led to the death of the woman *(27)*. Furthermore, the interviewer's level of competence in collecting information and the ability of health care workers or algorithms to determine the diagnosis from the history of an illness prior to death add to the potential for inaccuracy in diagnoses. Reports on the characteristic symptoms of a death have been shown to become more vague with passing time, making the classification of cause of death more difficult *(25)*.

More information on verbal autopsy techniques can be found in the MEASURE Evaluation Compendium of Maternal and Newborn Health Tools (www.cpc.unc.edu/measure/cmnht/cmnht.html).

Qualitative Research

In terms of maternal health, qualitative research attempts to understand how cultural and social experiences shape health-related phenomena. The word *qualitative* implies a focus on processes and meanings that are not always examined or measured in terms of quantity, amount, intensity, or frequency. Instead, qualitative research uses approaches that are shaped by and are relevant to the social context of women's lives to measure the level of reproductive mortality and morbidity in a society.

Attempting to Learn About Maternal
Health in Bangladesh

The maternal mortality ratio in Bangladesh is among the highest in the world, about 600 deaths per 100,000 live births (28), and recent studies conducted in Bangladesh suggest that the number of acute maternal morbidities may be as high as 67 episodes for every maternal death (29). Even in light of these alarming estimates, few published data exist on postpartum morbidity, experiences of illness during the puerperium, or local beliefs and customs relating to postpartum morbidity.

In December 1991, researchers at the Research and Evaluation Division of the Bangladesh Rural Advancement Committee (BRAC) undertook a prospective study of postpartum morbidity and its relation to delivery practices. The main objectives of the study were to determine the nature and incidence of illness during the puerperium and to define the risk factors for morbidity. Researchers devised three types of focus groups to obtain a comprehensive picture of experiences and opinions on sensitive issues surrounding maternal health within the community: 1) young, less experienced mothers; 2) older, more experienced mothers; and 3) traditional birth attendants, both trained and untrained. The three main topics of discussion were beliefs about disease causation and prevention during pregnancy and the puerperium, delivery practices and experiences of childbirth, and postpartum health problems.

By the completion of the study in June 1993, more than 1,500 women had participated in the focus group discussions. A significant finding from this study was an unmet need for basic postpartum health care available to village women. Although a wide range of locally available treatments exists, knowledge of antibiotics in treatment, for example, is rare. Another finding was that mothers and TBAs had very similar belief systems in terms of disease causation and the proper practices to follow. This discovery has implications on the impact of TBAs as a force of change in the care of pregnant and parturient women—if TBAs themselves do not believe a change in customs will be beneficial, they will not be able to convince mothers. Perhaps most significantly, these discussions revealed major differences between the model of disease causation and treatment used by health workers and the knowledge of local women and TBAs. Many of the Western concepts of antenatal care for a normal pregnancy and of risk detection or preventive care used by medical practitioners were alien to the women in the study. Due to a lack of health education and the highly medicalized nature of pregnancy services, the preventive aspect of modern antenatal care had not been incorporated into the women's belief system. Researchers suggested that the identification and encouragement of the use of beneficial local customs and beliefs are likely to improve the relationship between local communities and formal medical services and, thus, improve maternal health in Bangladesh.

Because the health of a woman is so entwined in the social and behavioral aspects of her surroundings, qualitative approaches have an important role in maternal health research. This form of research, quite different from quantitative research, seeks to understand and interpret personal experiences, cultural practices, behaviors, and health care utilization to explain health-related phenomena. Despite the differences, an important link exists between the two types of research. Often, qualitative research precedes quantitative research as a useful means of targeting what type of quantitative research should be conducted. For example, the information generated through qualitative focus groups may help in the formulation of questions that can be incorporated into household surveys. In many instances, qualitative research can address questions that quantitative research cannot, such as why women do not adhere to a health care regimen or why a certain health care intervention succeeds or fails.

Qualitative research makes use of many methods of data collection, including case studies, participant observation, focus groups and in-depth interviews, and several approaches to data analysis. Regarding maternal health, information is needed not only about the disease conditions from which women suffer, but also about the social determinants of these conditions. For this reason, qualitative research is increasingly being recognized as an important tool in the area of maternal health research. In many cases, this form of research may provide important insights into health-related phenomena and can guide further research questions.

The following text is recommended for further details on qualitative methods:

Patton MQ. Qualitative evaluation and research methods. 2nd ed. Newbury Park (CA): Sage Publications; 1990.

EPIDEMIOLOGIC STUDIES

Once the highest priority problems have been identified through the examination of surveillance, vital statistics, and other descriptive data, each problem must be analyzed in order to understand its causes, consequences, and strengths of the relationship between them. In some situations, the data collected through large-scale demographic surveys are useful for assessing priority areas in maternal health. Epidemiologic studies are then used to test specific hypotheses raised by these large-scale demographic studies. However, if data of acceptable quality are not available, the next step is to consider collecting the primary data through epidemiologic studies.

Epidemiologic studies are classified as either descriptive or analytic, depending on the primary purpose of the research. *Descriptive studies* are used to attain additional information necessary to make specific hypotheses. They provide baseline data on the occurrence or prevalence of a characteristic related to a health event and information on the people affected by the health event (see "An Epidemiologic Approach to Reproductive Health," chapter 6 on descriptive studies). *Analytic studies* are used to investigate associations between risk factors and outcomes by testing specific causal hypotheses (see "An Epidemiologic Approach to Reproductive Health," chapters 8–10 on randomized clinical trials, and cohort and case-control studies).

Once the purpose of the research has been decided, the process of developing the study plan can begin. Beyond the purpose of the study, choosing its design is based on several factors, including cost, and the nature of the population and variables to be studied. Although other types of analytic studies exist, this discussion will be limited to cohort and case-control studies.

Assessing Risk Factors for Maternal Mortality in Three Main Hospitals in Dakar, Senegal

Researchers in Senegal noticed that a large proportion of maternal deaths in Senegal were occurring in hospitals and became interested in determining the major risk factors associated with maternal deaths occurring in the three main hospitals of Dakar, the capital city (30). They identified 152 maternal deaths over a 12-month period and matched each of these cases with two controls on the basis of age, birth order, and place and time of delivery. The leading causes of death in these cases were puerperal sepsis (51 cases), hemorrhage (32 cases), eclampsia (29 cases), ruptured uterus (11 cases), and anemia (7 cases).

Results of the study revealed that the major risk factors for maternal deaths associated with failures at the hospitals were medical equipment failure (odds ratio [OR]=55.0), late referral (OR=23.2), lack of antenatal visit (OR=16.9), and lack of available personnel at time of admission (OR=6.6). Besides hospital failures, other correlates of maternal mortality included being unmarried (OR=2.5), rainy season (OR=2.4), first pregnancy (OR=2.3), pregnancy of high birth order (1.9), and low level of education (OR=1.6). These results have important implications for hospital policy: the identification of risk factors may lead to changes in health planning and resource allocation that could significantly affect the number of maternal deaths in this setting.

Cohort Studies

In the cohort design, investigators identify a population (cohort) and determine its initial characteristics or risk factors (exposure). The subjects are then followed over time to measure the outcome of interest in the exposed and unexposed groups. The temporal aspect of this design makes it possible for the investigator to describe the incidence of the outcomes in the cohort.

The cohort study can be conducted either prospectively or retrospectively. The prospective cohort design is a powerful strategy for defining the incidence and investigating the potential causes of a health event. Measuring current levels of the predictor variables *before the outcome occurs* generally produces more accurate data than attempts to reconstruct past exposures after the outcome has already happened. For example, if maternal deaths are studied retrospectively, it would

---

Assessing Neonatal Outcomes Associated With Placenta Previa in Nova Scotia, Canada

Placenta previa is a major cause of antepartum hemorrhage, estimated to occur in 0.31% to 0.60% of pregnancies at delivery (31). In this condition, excessive bleeding occurs due to the separation of a placenta whose position in the uterus is abnormal, usually attached partly or entirely to the inner surface of the lower part of the uterus. To identify neonatal complications associated with placenta previa, researchers in the Canadian province of Nova Scotia conducted a population-based retrospective cohort study involving all singleton deliveries from 1988 to 1995. Information was collected from the Nova Scotia Atlee Perinatal Database and was then coded using a system modified from the International Classification of Diseases for variables including maternal and neonatal outcomes, details of medical histories, and sociodemographic characteristics. The study group comprised all completed singleton pregnancies complicated by placenta previa, and all other singleton pregnancies were considered controls. Of the 92,983 women who delivered singletons during the 8 years of the study, 305 births were coded for placenta previa, a prevalence of 0.33%.

Previous studies have suggested associations between placenta previa and preterm birth, low birth weight, congenital anomalies, respiratory depression at birth, respiratory distress syndrome, intraventricular hemorrhage, anemia, and low Apgar scores, but these studies had not adjusted for maternal age. In this study, after adjusting for potential confounders, the significant neonatal complications for women with placenta previa included major congenital anomalies (odds ratio [OR]=2.48), respiratory distress syndrome (OR=4.94), and anemia (OR=2.65). This study also confirmed that preterm birth, admission to neonatal intensive care unit, and length of neonatal hospital stay were significantly increased in pregnancies complicated by placenta previa. The association between placenta previa and perinatal mortality was not significant. This study took place in a setting where techniques such as transvaginal ultrasound, maternal steroids for lung maturity, and neonatal surfactants were available. Because this study incorporated current obstetric practices, knowledge of complications of placenta previa can be used to improve prenatal counseling and neonatal treatment in this setting.

be necessary to reconstruct past predictor variables from medical records or other sources, such as friends and relatives of the deceased women. The prospective cohort design also prevents measurements from being biased by knowledge of the outcome. In the retrospective cohort design, on the other hand, the assembly of the cohort, baseline measurements, follow-up, and outcomes all happened in the past. This type of study is possible when data about the risk factors and outcomes are available for a cohort of subjects assembled for other purposes.

The main weakness of the prospective cohort study is that it is an expensive, and often inefficient, way to study risk factors for the occurrence of a health event. Even for relatively common outcomes, large numbers of subjects must be followed for long periods of time to produce meaningful results. Another problem with the retrospective cohort design is that the investigator has no control over the nature and quality of the measurements that are made. In some instances, the existing data may not include information important to answering the research question. Or, if the existing data do include the relevant information, they may be incomplete, inaccurate, or measured in a way that is not optimal for answering the research question.

Case-Control Studies

With the exception of the most common diseases, cohort studies are expensive and require large sample sizes to identify risk factors for relatively rare diseases. For most risk factors, a reference group must be assembled so that the prevalence of the risk factor in subjects with the condition (case subjects) can be compared with that of subjects without the condition (control subjects). This study design, called a case-control study, identifies groups of subjects as cases and controls and then looks back in time to find differences in predictor variables that may explain why the case subjects became ill and the control subjects did not. Case-control studies are generally retrospective; however, this study design can also be used prospectively; that is, cases and controls are enrolled in the study soon after the health event is identified. Case-control studies are especially useful if the outcome is a rare event.

Case-control studies provide descriptive information on the characteristics of cases as well as an estimate of the strength of the association between each predictor variable and the presence or absence of the disease in the form of an odds ratio. One of the major strengths of case-control studies is their high yield of information from relatively few subjects. For health events that are rare or have long latent periods between exposure and disease, a case-control study is far more efficient than a cohort study and is often the only feasible option. The retrospective approach of a case-control study makes it

What Is Causing Maternal Mortality in Maharashtra State, India?

More than a decade after the launch of the global Safe Motherhood Initiative in 1987, maternal deaths in India still account for 13% of all deaths among women of reproductive age (32). National estimates of maternal mortality range from 4 to 5.5 per 1000 live births; however, they differ significantly between urban and rural areas. In the rural regions of the state of Maharashtra, where maternal mortality ratios have been variously estimated as 3.3 and 2.16 per 1000 live births, researchers became interested in determining the main causes of maternal deaths.

Researchers conducted a population-based, matched case-control study to compare women who died of pregnancy-related causes with women who had similar biomedical complications but survived. All deaths of women aged 15–45 years were identified using multiple sources, such as vital registration records, primary health center registers, surveillance of public and private medical facilities, and an informal "village information system" composed of women's groups, community health volunteers, and school teachers. One hundred twenty-one maternal deaths (cases) were enrolled prospectively from January to December 1995, and two controls per case were drawn from the same population base as the cases.

The data were collected using a structured interview and history taken from the husband's family and the wife's own family, interviews with health care providers, and a review of available medical records. Results of the study revealed that direct obstetric causes accounted for 71.9% of the maternal deaths; the main causes were postpartum hemorrhage (30.6%), puerperal sepsis (13.2%), eclampsia (8.3%), and anemia (5.8%). Adjusted odds ratios indicated a negative effect of excessive referrals (OR=2.24) and a protective effect of residing in the village (OR=0.36), presence of a resident nurse in the village (OR=0.42), having an educated husband (OR=0.46), and the presence of a trained attendant at delivery (OR=0.49). On the basis of this study, interventions such as changing the health care referral structure or ensuring the presence of a trained birth attendant may have strong influences in reducing maternal mortality in this setting.

a useful tool for examining a large number of predictive variables and for generating hypotheses about the causes of health events. The benefits of case-control studies are achieved at a cost. The information that can be obtained using case-control studies is limited—the incidence or prevalence of the health event cannot be directly estimated because the proportion of those with the condition is determined not by their proportion in the population, but by how many cases and controls the investigator chooses to sample. Because risk factors may vary for different causes of maternal mortality, conducting general case-control studies is not always helpful in determining associations between hypothesized risk factors and the outcome. Perhaps the biggest weakness of case-control studies is their susceptibility to bias resulting from the separate sampling of cases and controls, and the retrospective measurement of the predictor variables.

IMPLICATIONS OF RESEARCH AND COLLECTED DATA

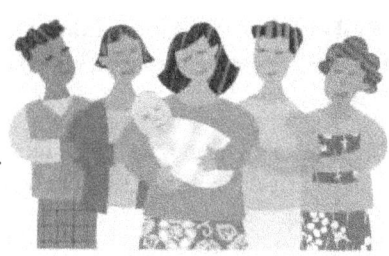

The methods described above are mechanisms for providing information that can be used to guide public health efforts in reducing maternal mortality. The regular and systematic collection of data allows maternal health events in a population to be compared with an expected value. Assessment of this data may point to particular areas that could benefit from further research. The last step, perhaps the most crucial, is to communicate the results in a manner that will help lead to a measurable improvement in the current maternal health situation.

Comparing the observed data to an expected value is critical to evaluate the acceptability of the current maternal health situation. This comparison transforms the data into useful *information*. Information is an indispensable tool for health care workers; it may be used to focus the attention of decision makers on the problem of maternal mortality and morbidity, refine current health programs, and guide planning for future programs to lessen the burden of deaths and disability due to maternal causes. The following story illustrates how strides were made in reducing maternal mortality in Cuba when routinely collected data were transformed into information useful to health workers and policymakers.

The Ministry of Public Health of Cuba decided in 1962 to investigate every death related to pregnancy, delivery, and the puerperium *(33)*. Whenever possible, a case was investigated by a specialist not previously involved with it, such as a doctor from outside the hospital where the death occurred. This procedure offered the greatest likelihood of determining the cause of death and any unfavorable attendant circumstances. Group discussions of the circumstances leading to the deaths of these women provided educational opportunities where shortcomings in medical care were highlighted. Out of this study and discussions arose the national application of obstetric standards in Cuba.

Results of this routine data collection indicate a large drop in Cuba's maternal mortality—compared with 1962, maternal mortality was about 75% lower at the end of the study in 1984. Table 3 indicates the main causes of maternal deaths.

The most striking changes have been in deaths from toxemia, which fell from 35 to under 4 per 100,000 live births between 1960 and 1984, and in deaths from hemorrhage, which fell from 32 to under 2 per 100,000 live births in the same interval. The decrease in deaths

Table 3. Causes of Maternal Deaths* in Cuba, 1960–1984

Causes	1960	1970	1975	1980	1984
Toxemia of pregnancy and the puerperium	35	6	11	4	4
Hemorrhage of pregnancy and childbirth	32	8	6	6	2
Abortion	14	22	12	15	5
Sepsis of childbirth and the puerperium	9	8	12	9	6
Other complications of pregnancy, childbirth, and the puerperium	29	28	27	19	15

*Maternal deaths per 100,000 live births.
Source: Farnot Cardoso U. Giving birth is safer now. World Health Forum 1986;7:348–52.

from toxemia is attributed to improved antenatal care and improved socioeconomic and nutritional conditions. The increase in the proportion of births in large hospitals, where medical surveillance is continuous and blood banks are available for emergencies, has contributed to the decline in deaths from hemorrhage. Also, the decline in deaths from abortions in the more recent years is a result of the policy of providing facilities in hospitals for the interruption of unwanted pregnancies.

How Should the Data Be Presented to Best Communicate the Results of the Analysis?

"Good" data are those that are reliable and presented in a way that is easily understood by all who need to know. The selection of the data presentation format should be based on two main factors: the purpose of the analysis and the audience for whom it is intended. Maternal health data can be analyzed by time, place, and person to formulate outcome and process indicators useful for detecting trends in particular health events, monitoring existing health programs, and assessing risk factors.

The results of the analysis need to be adequately presented to achieve the intended objectives. The information can be presented in several ways—perhaps the most effective way is through graphs, maps, and tables to enhance the impact of the information at a glance. Depending on the resources of the particular area, available channels of communication may include chalkboards, posters and pamphlets, publications, electronic media (for example, telecommunications systems, fax machines, audio and video conferences), mass media, and public forums. Regardless of the media, a clear, concise, visual style of presentation is generally the most effective means of communicating the information. Ultimately, the effective communication of maternal health information is the critical link in translating scientific information into public health practice.

Who Needs to Know the Results of the Research, and Why?

Interpreting and communicating the results are the next steps in the process of transforming the data into information for action. Good data play a crucial role in allowing health staff to modify and refine the way they are doing things in the field, and also in focusing the attention of policymakers on the current maternal health situation. Therefore, those who need to know the findings include those who are the source of the primary data (such as health care providers and laboratory personnel) as well as those who are involved in administrative or program planning, and decision making.

Results and recommendations serve to inform and motivate health personnel, who are more likely to continue the challenging job of collecting information if they know that it is being used and acted on. This same type of feedback is important between the regional and national levels; for example, a need for training or resources at the local level may be identified, which is available only from the regional level. This communication may be facilitated through periodic meetings at the regional and national levels.

How Are the Data Turned Into Action That Will Help Improve Maternal Health?

It is critical that the results and recommendations generated by the data lead to concrete action for achieving the objectives of the maternal health program. Interventions may take place at all levels of the health care system—community, formal health care system, and intersectoral—and include changes in the outlook, knowledge, skills and resources of the system. The data should be used to develop feasible, effective, and efficient strategies for reducing maternal mortality and morbidity. Developed by WHO in 1994, the Mother-Baby Package *(6)* outlines strategies for simple and cost-effective interventions that should significantly improve maternal health.

What Is the Purpose of Evaluating Existing Maternal Health Programs?

To assess the degree to which a health program is achieving its goals and targets, a system for monitoring and evaluation must be established. Regular review of a maternal health program allows health staff to modify and refine health actions taking place in the field. Evaluation is an important step in promoting the best use of public health resources and should include recommendations for improving quality and efficiency. Most importantly, an evaluation should assess whether the program is serving a useful public health function and is meeting its overall objective of reducing maternal mortality and morbidity.

Evaluation generally involves the definition of indicators to track progress toward explicit objectives. Once the objectives of a maternal health program have been defined, indicators are used as markers of progress toward reducing maternal mortality and morbidity. The indicator can either be a direct measure of outcomes or may indirectly measure progress toward specified process goals. An indicator can be thought of as a measurement that provides information regarding a health outcome, when compared with a standard or desired level of achievement. The calculation of these indicators can be repeated over time as a measure of progress.

In summary, the goals of evaluation are to

• Select appropriate interventions that reflect local needs.

• Build on lessons learned and programs that have worked in other countries.

• Implement interventions according to current best practices.

• Monitor their progress.

Evaluation can be used to guide future programming and help us reach goals set for improving maternal health *(26)*.

REFERENCES

1. Juncker T, Khan M, Ahmed S. Interventions in obstetric care: lessons learned from Abhoynagar. Working Paper No. 124. Dhaka: International Centre for Diarrhoeal Disease Research, Bangladesh (ICDDR,B); 1996.

2. AbouZahr C. Maternal mortality overview. In: Murray CJL, Lopez AD, editors. Health dimensions of sex and reproduction. Boston: Harvard University Press; 1998. p. 111–64.

3. Royston E, Armstrong S, editors. Preventing maternal deaths. London: World Health Organization; 1989.

4. CDC. Maternal mortality—United States, 1982–1996. MMWR 1998;47(34):705–7.

5. Kao S, Chen LM, Shi L, Weinrich MC. Underreporting and misclassification of maternal mortality in Taiwan. Acta Obstet Gynecol Scand 1997;76(7):629–36.

6. World Health Organization. Mother-baby package: implementing safe motherhood in countries. Rev. ed. Geneva, Switzerland: World Health Organization, Maternal Health and Safe Motherhood Programme, Division of Family Health; 1996.

7. DHS Analytical Report No. 4. DHS maternal mortality indicators: an assessment of data quality and implications for data use. Calverton (MD): Macro International, Inc.; 1997.

8. Zurayk H, Khattab H, Younis N, El-Mouelhy M, Fadle M. Reproductive health and reproductive morbidity: concepts and measures with relevance to Middle Eastern society. In: Boerma JT, editor. Measurement of maternal and child mortality, morbidity, and health care. Belgium: Derouaux Ordina Editions; 1992. p. 225–59.

9. World Health Organization. WHO revised 1990 estimates of maternal mortality: a new approach by WHO and UNICEF. Geneva, Switzerland: World Health Organization; 1996. p. 1–15.

10. World Health Organization. Coverage of maternity care: a tabulation of available information. 3rd edition. Geneva, Switzerland: World Health Organization, Maternal Health and Safe Motherhood Programme, Division of Family Health; 1993.

11. Dietz PM, Rochat RW, Thompson BL, Berg CJ, Griffin GW. Differences in the risk of homicide and other fatal injuries between postpartum women and other women of childbearing age: implications for prevention. Am J Public Health 1998;88(4):641–3.

12. World Health Organization/The World Bank. Maternal health around the world [poster]. Washington: World Health Organization and The World Bank; 1997.

13. DeSilva WI. Puerperal morbidity: a neglected area of maternal health in Sri Lanka. Soc Biol 1998;45(3–4):223–45.

14. Mantel GD, Buchmann E, Rees H, Pattinson RC. Severe acute maternal morbidity: a pilot study of a definition for a near-miss. Br J Obstet Gynaecol 1998;105:985–90.

15. World Health Organization. Maternal mortality: a global factbook. Geneva, Switzerland: World Health Organization; 1991.

16. Berg C, Danel I, Mora G, editors. Guidelines for maternal mortality epidemiological surveillance. Washington: The World Bank; 1996.

17. Safe motherhood indicators—lessons learned in measuring progress. MotherCare Matters 1999;8:1–24.

18. Danel I. Keeping our eyes on the target—the importance of monitoring maternal mortality. MotherCare Matters 1999;8:2–3.

19. The EVALUATION Project. Indicators for reproductive health program evaluation: final report of the subcommittee on safe pregnancy. Chapel Hill (NC): Carolina Population Center, University of North Carolina; 1995.

20. World Health Organization. Reduction of maternal mortality. A joint WHO/UNFPA/UNICEF World Bank Statement. Geneva, Switzerland: World Health Organization; 1999.

21. Le Coeur S, Pictet G, M'Pele P, Lallemant M. Direct estimation of maternal mortality in Africa. Lancet 1998;352(9139):1525–26.

22. Serbanescu F, Morris L, Stupp P, Stanescu A. The impact of recent policy changes on fertility, abortion, and contraceptive use in Romania. Stud Fam Plan 1995;26(2):76–87.

23. Stephenson P, Wagner M, Badea M, Serbanescu F. Commentary: the public health consequences of restricted induced abortion—lessons from Romania. Am J Public Health 1992;82(10):1328–31.

24. Danel I, Graham W, Stupp P, Castillo P. Applying the sisterhood method for estimating maternal mortality to a health facility-based sample: a comparison with results from a household-based sample. Int J Epidemiol 1996;25(5):1017–22.

25. Høj L, Stensballe J, Aaby P. Maternal mortality in Guinea–Bissau: the use of verbal autopsy in a multi-ethnic population. Int J Epidemiol 1999;28:70–6.

26. CARE. Promoting quality maternal and newborn care: a reference manual for program managers. Atlanta (GA): Cooperative for Assistance and Relief Everywhere; 1998.

27. Chandramohan D, Rodrigues L, Maude G, Hayes R. The validity of verbal autopsies for assessing the causes of institutional maternal death. Stud Fam Plan 1998;29(4):414–22.

28. Goodburn EA, Gazi R, Chowdhury M. Beliefs and practices regarding delivery and postpartum maternal morbidity in rural Bangladesh. Stud Fam Plan 1995;26(1):22–32.

29. Koblinsky MA, Campbell OMR, Harlow S. Mother and more: a broader perspective on women's health. In: Koblinsky MA, Timyan J, Gay J, editors. The health of women: a global perspective. Boulder (CO): Westview Press; 1993.

30. Garenne M, Mbaye K, Bah M, Correa P. Risk factors for maternal mortality: a case-control study in Dakar hospitals (Senegal). Afr J Reprod Health 1997;1(1):14–24.

31. Crane JMG, Van den Hof MC, Dodds L, Armson BA, Liston R. Neonatal outcomes with placenta previa. Obstet Gynecol 1999;93(4):541–4.

32. Ganatra BR, Coyaji KJ, Rao VN. Too far, too little, too late: a community-based case-control study of maternal mortality in rural west Maharashtra, India. World Health Organ 1998;76(6):591–8.

33. Farnot Cardoso U. Giving birth is safer now. World Health Forum 1986;7:348–52.

CASE STUDY: MATERNAL MORTALITY IN EGYPT

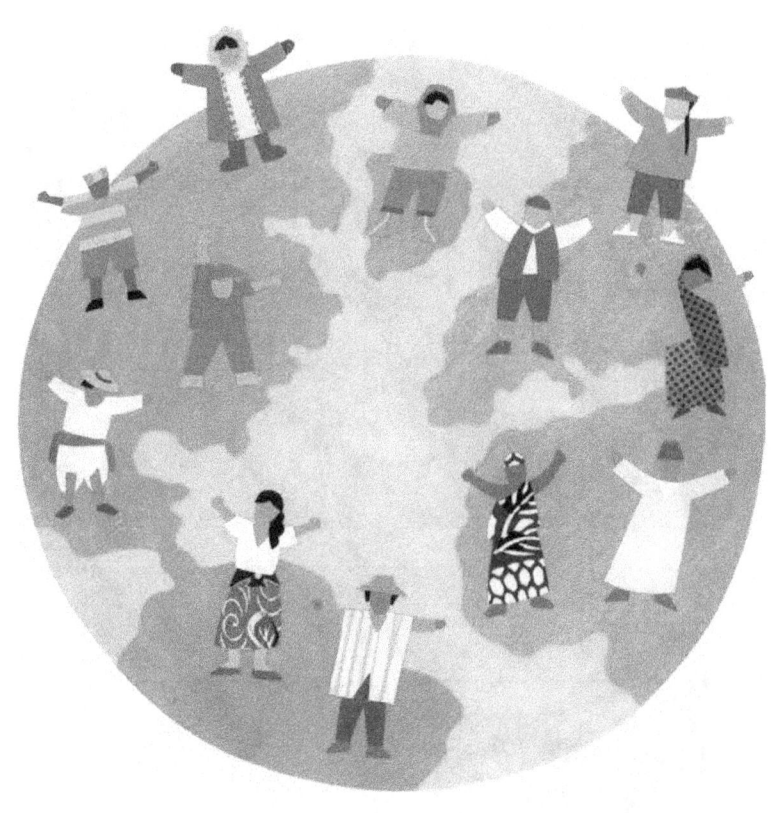

CASE STUDY: MATERNAL MORTALITY IN EGYPT[†]

Introduction

In 1992, the Ministry of Health of Egypt began the first national study of maternal mortality. The main goal of this study was to gather information useful in the development of programs and policies to decrease maternal deaths in Egypt.

Q1: If you were planning a national study of maternal mortality, what might you include as the specific objectives of the study?

Study Design and Methods

The National Maternal Mortality Study: Egypt, 1992–1993, was the first national study of maternal mortality conducted in Egypt. Launched by the Ministry of Health, the objectives of this study were

- To obtain a national figure of maternal mortality in Egypt.
- To identify the main causes of maternal mortality.
- To determine the avoidable factors contributing to these maternal deaths.
- To develop preventive programs to reduce maternal mortality.

The National Maternal Mortality Study is a population-based sample of all maternal deaths that occurred over a 1-year period in 21 governorates of Egypt. Within these governorates, a random sample of 122 health bureaus was drawn, which includes approximately 28% of all registered deaths of females of reproductive age (14–50 years) in Egypt. A maternal mortality study committee, called the Local Advisory Group (LAG), was formed in each governorate. Each LAG was chaired by the Undersecretary of Health in that governorate, and consisted of three senior obstetricians. The sample size was determined to provide precise estimates of the maternal mortality ratio for three strata: upper, lower, and metropolitan Egypt.

Each week, the selected health bureaus received notification of deaths from different health bureaus in its area. Deaths of women between the ages of 14 and 50 years were identified by the directors of the selected health bureaus for a 1-year period beginning March 1, 1992. Among these deaths, maternal deaths were initially identified by a screening questionnaire at the health bureaus. The director of the selected health bureau visited the household where the death occurred to determine whether the deceased was pregnant or died within 42 days of delivery or abortion. If the death was

---

[†]Adapted from: Egypt Ministry of Health. National maternal mortality study: Egypt, 1992–1993. Findings and conclusions. Cairo, Egypt: Child Survival Project; 1994.

determined to be due to maternal causes, the LAG was notified. The LAG then notified professional social workers at the governorate level, who collected information on these deaths through an in-depth home interview with the closest relatives of the deceased woman. If a traditional birth attendant was involved, she was also interviewed by the social worker.

All questionnaires were then sent back to the LAG. If the deceased woman had been taken to a physician or health facility, the medical records were reviewed and health care practitioners interviewed by LAG obstetricians. Other sources of information included midwives involved in the care of the woman, any person who witnessed the death, drug and x-ray prescription forms, and medical records from MCH units, hospitals, or private clinics. All questionnaires and records were reviewed, causes of death were assigned by consensus, and avoidable factors were evaluated. The LAGs sent all questionnaires and technical documents to the Central Advisory Group (CAG) for review and finalization.

The CAG is responsible for coding and entering questionnaires, analyzing the data, and disseminating the results. The CAG also organizes training for selected health bureau directors and LAGs and provides refresher courses. Information from this study will be used by the Minister of Health, senior policymakers, eminent members of the medical profession (including deans of medical schools, obstetricians, anesthetists, and professors of community medicine), and international donors to implement programs to reduce maternal mortality in Egypt.

Exercises

Q2: Draw a simple sketch of the flow of information in the National Maternal Mortality Study.

Q3: What are the steps in determining the number of maternal deaths due to direct and indirect causes?

Q4: Table 1 shows data on female deaths (FD), maternal deaths (MD), and the maternal mortality ratio (MMR) in three strata of Egypt, as well as for the total study area:

Previous studies have shown that in developing countries with high maternal mortality, between one-quarter and one-third of female deaths are usually due to maternal causes (Royston and Armstrong, 1989). Look at the percentage of female deaths that were maternal deaths (MD/FD) for the total study area. How does this percentage compare with MD/FD in other developing countries?

Table 1. Female Deaths, Maternal Deaths, and Maternal Mortality, by Strata

Strata	Live Births	FD	MD	MD/FD	MMR
Metropolitan	60,882	1,702	142	8.3	233
Lower Egypt	237,006	3,564	314	8.8	132
Upper Egypt	145,360	2,221	316	14.2	217
Total Area	443,248	7,487	772	10.3	174

Notes: FD=female deaths, MD=maternal deaths, MMR=maternal mortality ratio

Suggest some reasons for why MD/FD is lower than expected, compared with other developing countries.

In terms of level of socioeconomic development, metropolitan Egypt ranks highest, followed by lower Egypt and, lastly, upper Egypt. Given this information, is the pattern of female deaths due to maternal causes what you would expect it to be?

Q5: There is evidence that the level of fertility in Egypt has declined from past levels (DHS II: Egypt, 1993). Which statistics would be affected by a decrease in fertility: the maternal mortality ratio (MMR), the maternal mortality rate, or both? Why?

Q6: It is generally accepted that the youngest and oldest mothers are at greatest risk of dying from pregnancy-related causes. Table 2 illustrates the frequency in this study of maternal mortality and percentage of women giving birth, by age group.

Table 2. Frequency of Maternal Mortality and Percentage of Women Giving Birth, by Age Group

Age Group	Number of Maternal Deaths	Percentage of Maternal Deaths	Percentage of Women Giving Birth
<20	29	4.0	6.3
20–24	101	14.1	20.8
25–29	165	23.0	22.2
30–34	152	21.2	15.5
35–39	182	25.3	8.9
40+	89	12.4	2.5
Total	**718**	**100.0**	**76.2**

Source: Egypt DHS II (1993).

Given this information, do you recommend targeting preventive approaches toward women in the youngest (<20) and oldest (40+) age groups as an effective way of reducing maternal mortality in this setting? Why or why not?

Q7: Table 3 shows data on the outcome for the fetus or infant, by time of death of the mother:

Table 3. Outcome for the Fetus or Infant, by Time of Death of the Mother

Outcome	Number of Maternal Deaths	Percentage of Maternal Deaths
Mother and fetus died in early pregnancy	87	12.1
Mother and fetus died undelivered	95	13.2
Mother died in delivery		
Infant alive	157	21.9
Infant dead	124	17.3
Mother died postpartum		
Infant alive	151	21.0
Infant dead	<u>104</u>	<u>14.5</u>
Total	**718**	**100.0**

Of the 718 maternal deaths for which questionnaires were completed, what percentage of the fetuses/infants also died?

What does this percentage tell us about the effects of maternal deaths on child survival in Egypt?

Q8: The term avoidable factor, sometimes called substandard care, takes into account failures in clinical care and also some of the underlying factors that may have produced a low standard of care for women, including patient, family, and situational factors. The examination of avoidable factors that contribute to maternal death is an important step in designing and implementing prevention programs.

List some avoidable factors that may contribute to maternal deaths.

Table 4 provides data on the avoidable factors contributing to maternal deaths in this study:

Table 4. Selected Avoidable Factors in Relation to Maternal Deaths

Factor	Total*	
	No.	**%**
No or poor quality ANC	239	33
Delay in seeking medical care	304	42
Unwanted pregnancy	36	5
Substandard care from		
General practitioner	87	12
Obstetric team	334	47
Daya (TBA)	84	12
Lack of blood bank	45	6
Cause of death could have been detected during ANC	341	47
No avoidable factors	54	8

Notes: daya=traditional birth attendant, ANC=Antenatal care.
*Total includes deaths due to direct, indirect, and unknown causes; percentages do not add up to 100% because each death may have more than one avoidable factor.

What percentage of the maternal deaths were felt to be unavoidable with standard level of care, and what does this percentage imply about the remaining maternal deaths?

What were found to be the leading avoidable factors resulting in maternal deaths? Which of these factors were health facility factors, and which were patient factors?

Q9: Consider the following table of characteristics of the maternal deaths in this study:

Table 5. Characteristics of Maternal Deaths

	All Deaths (N=718)	
	n	%
Antenatal care		
Never	249	35
1 or 2	107	15
3 or more	359	50
Missing data	3	0
Place of delivery		
None	182	25
Home	213	30
Public facility	239	33
Private facility	84	12

Surprisingly, these results suggest that women who attended antenatal care the most frequently and women who delivered in a public facility were slightly more likely to die. What is a possible explanation for these findings?

Q10: Cause-specific results are an important way of determining whether a given factor plays a particular role in contributing to mortality from that cause. In total, of 718 maternal deaths, 499 were due to direct causes and 193 were due to indirect causes (the causes of the remaining 26 deaths were unknown). Table 6 presents selected data on avoidable factors for cause-specific deaths.

Table 6. Summary of Avoidable Factors for Cause-Specific Deaths*

		Hemorrhage			
Causes	All N=718	Antepartum N=58	Postpartum N=178	Hypertension N=114	Sepsis N=60
Avoidable causes					
ANC-related**	239 (33%)	32 (55%)	40 (22%)	59 (52%)	10 (17%)
Delay	304 (42%)	35 (60%)	62 (35%)	64 (56%)	18 (30%)
Substandard care					
General practitioner	87 (12%)	5 (9%)	14 (8%)	8 (7%)	10 (17%)
Obstetric team	334 (47%)	33 (57%)	110 (62%)	71 (62%)	21 (35%)
Daya	84 (12%)	6 (10%)	42 (24%)	2 (2%)	22 (37%)
Shortages					
Blood	45 (6%)	8 (14%)	36 (20%)	1 (1%)	0
Transportation/distance	28 (4%)	0	0	2 (2%)	0
Drug supply/equipment	15 (2%)	5 (9%)	11 (6%)	3 (3%)	0
No avoidable factors	54 (8%)	1 (2%)	1 (1%)	1 (1%)	2 (3%)

	Abortion		Ruptured Uterus N=48	Cesarean Section N=44	Cardiac Disease N=55
Causes	Spontaneous N=19	Induced N=13			
Avoidable causes					
ANC-related**	4 (21%)	3 (23%)	16 (33%)	9 (20%)	24 (44%)
Delay	8 (42%)	3 (23%)	14 (29%)	10 (23%)	36 (65%)
Substandard care					
General practitioner	2 (11%)	0	4 (8%)	0	7 (13%)
Obstetric team	11 (58%)	10 (77%)	35 (73%)	41 (93%)	16 (29%)
Daya	0	0	6 (13%)	0	1 (2%)
Shortages					
Blood	1 (5%)	0	4 (8%)	5 (11%)	0
Transportation/distance	2 (11%)	0	2 (4%)	0	0
Drug supply/equipment	0	0	1 (2%)	5 (11%)	0
No avoidable factors	2 (11%)	0	0	0	4 (7%)

*Percents do not add up to 100, as there can be more than one direct cause.
**Both poor quality and inadequate attendance.

What were the top three causes of maternal deaths?

What percentage of all maternal deaths was associated with genital sepsis? What percentage of direct obstetric deaths was associated with genital sepsis?

What was the most commonly identified avoidable factor in sepsis-related deaths?

Substandard care by dayas (traditional birth attendants) was associated with 12% of all maternal deaths. Of these maternal deaths, 37% were related to genital sepsis, making dayas more likely to contribute to sepsis-related deaths than to other maternal deaths. Considering that nearly 70% of Egyptian women are delivered by a traditional birth attendant, what are the implications for the importance of interventions targeted at dayas in reducing maternal mortality?

Q11: On the basis of the results of this study, the following major conclusions were made:

a) Two major avoidable factors were revealed through the study—delays on the part of the woman and her family, and substandard care from medical professionals.

b) Substandard care on the part of obstetricians contributed to the deaths of nearly half the women (47%).

c) The study revealed that 70.6% of women attended a health facility at some point during the events leading to their deaths.

d) Many cases that resulted in hospital deaths were managed by junior obstetricians, or doctors-in-training, with limited experience.

e) Seventy percent of women are delivered by traditional birth attendants.

On the basis of these conclusions, can you suggest some potential recommendations?

Case Study: Maternal Mortality in Egypt
Answers

Q1: The purpose of the National Maternal Mortality Study was to gather information for developing programs that would decrease maternal mortality in Egypt. If you were planning a national study of maternal mortality, the specific objectives would be similar to those of the Egyptian study:

- To obtain a national figure of maternal mortality in Egypt.
- To identify the main causes of maternal mortality.
- To determine the avoidable factors contributing to these maternal deaths.
- To develop preventive programs to reduce maternal mortality.

Q2:

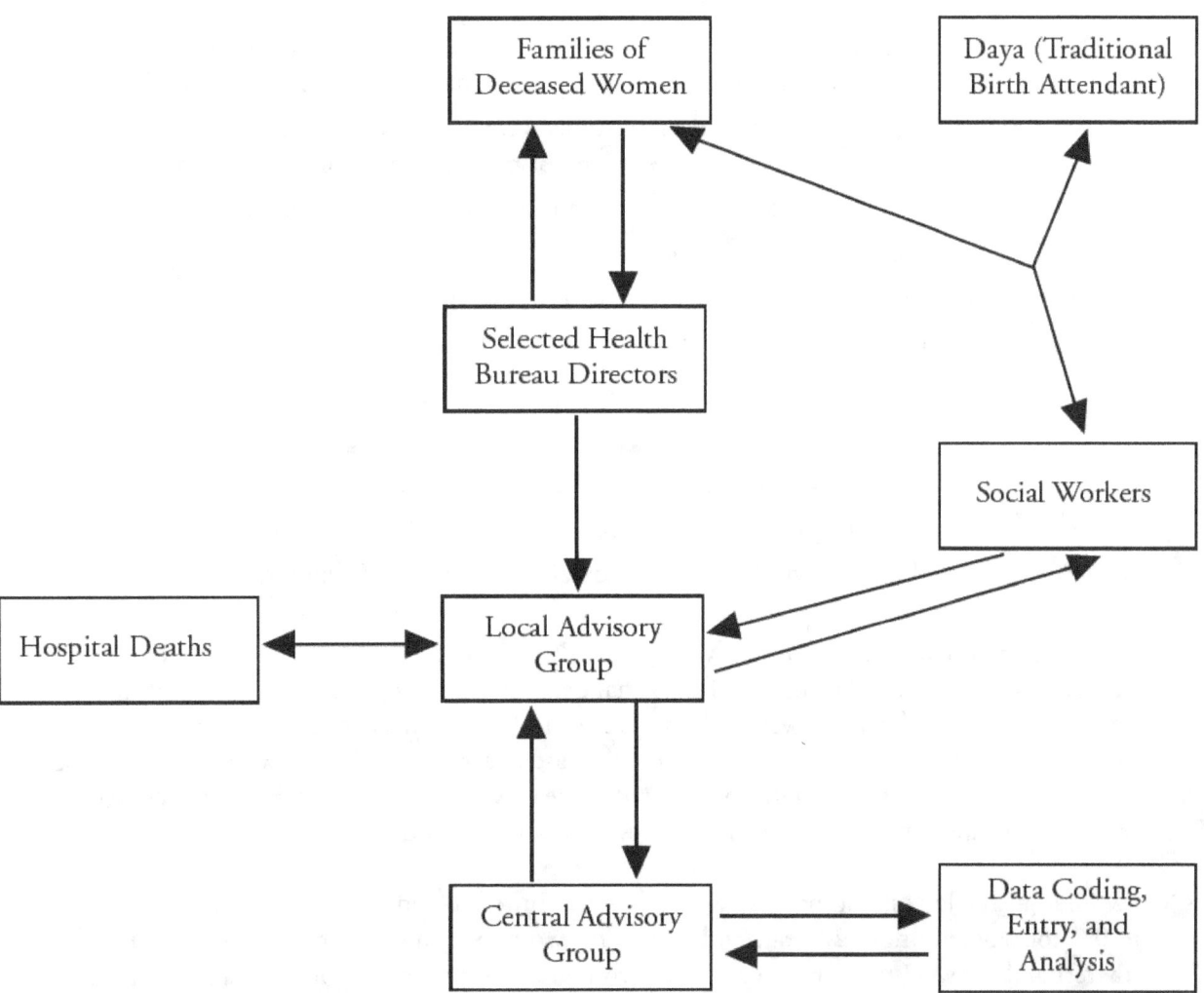

Q3:

- Identify all deaths of women of reproductive age (14–50 years, in this setting).
- Of these women, determine the number who died while pregnant, during delivery, or within the 42 days after the end of pregnancy. This is the number of maternal deaths due to all causes.
- Of these deaths, subtract the number of deaths due to incidental or accidental causes.
- The remainder is the number of maternal deaths due to direct and indirect causes.

Q4: In this study, the overall proportion of female deaths that were due to maternal causes (10.3%) is lower than expected. Previous studies have shown that between one-quarter and one-third of female deaths are usually due to maternal causes.

Several explanations why MD/FD is lower than expected, compared with other developing countries, are possible:

- Fertility has decreased in Egypt. A reduced number of pregnancies would reduce the number of maternal deaths and the percentage of female deaths due to maternal causes.
- The studies on which the expected proportions were based are outdated, and new studies should be done to get more accurate estimates of maternal mortality in developing countries.
- Maternal mortality in Egypt is lower than in other developing countries.
- Some maternal deaths may have been missed.

Generally, maternal deaths tend to decrease with increasing levels of development. The pattern of data from Egypt supports this trend:

Egyptian Strata	Level of Development	Maternal Deaths/ Female Deaths
Metro Egypt	Highest	8.3 (Lowest)
Lower Egypt	Medium	8.8 (Medium)
Upper Egypt	Lowest	14.2 (Highest)

Q5: Both the maternal mortality ratio (MMR) and the maternal mortality rate would be affected by the decrease in fertility. If the risk of maternal death remains constant, the maternal mortality rate will decrease, because fewer births will result in fewer maternal deaths. The MMR, on the other hand, may increase in an area with a decrease in fertility and no new safe motherhood interventions in place. A larger proportional decrease in the number of live births compared with the number of maternal deaths will result in an increased MMR.

Q6: Women in the lowest and highest age groups accounted for only 16.4% of maternal deaths—4.0% for women under 20 years and 12.4% for women aged 40 years and older. The bulk of maternal deaths, 83.6%, occurred among women between the ages of 20 and 39 years. Considering the percentage of women giving birth in the youngest and oldest age categories, preventive approaches focused on women defined as high risk based on age would not be the most effective way to reduce maternal mortality in this setting. Although these women have the highest risk of maternal death, they are the least likely to be pregnant. Instead, focusing preventive approaches on the ages of greatest likelihood of pregnancy (20–39) would help the greatest number of women and would be a more efficient use of the available resources.

Q7: Overall, 410 (87 + 95 + 124 + 104), or 57.1%, of the fetuses/infants of deceased women also died. If the mother died during delivery or the postpartum period, 228 (124 + 104), or 42.5%, of the infants died.

Previous research has shown that, after the death of a mother, the chances of survival for even older, living children of the deceased woman are significantly lowered. Overall, only about half of infants survived after the deaths of their mothers in this study. The chances of infant survival are slightly increased if the mother dies during childbirth or the postpartum period, compared with maternal deaths prior to delivery.

Q8: Avoidable factors may be classified as facility, medical team, or patient factors. The following are examples of avoidable factors:

Facility factors. Shortage of resources for staffing facilities, lack of transportation to facility, distance to nearest hospital, lack of blood bank, administrative failures in backup facilities (e.g., pathology, biochemistry, ultrasound, radiological services), and shortage or lack of drug availability (e.g., antibiotics, oxytocic drugs).

Medical team factors. Failure of diagnosis or management by general practitioner, obstetric team, or traditional birth attendant.

Patient and/or family factors. Delays in seeking medical care, noncompliance with medical care, or unwanted pregnancy.

Only 54 maternal deaths (8%) were felt to be unavoidable with standard-level care. In other words, at least one avoidable factor was identified for 92% of all maternal deaths in this study.

The leading avoidable factors were substandard care from the obstetric team (47%) and cause of death that could have been detected during antenatal care (47%). Delay in seeking medical care or noncompliance with medical care was another major contributor to maternal deaths (42%). No antenatal care or poor quality antenatal care contributed to 33% of maternal deaths. Major medical team and health facility factors include failure of early diagnosis and poor management (substandard care) by the obstetrician team, poor quality antenatal care, and cause of death that could have been detected during antenatal care. Patient factors include delay in seeking medical care or noncompliance with medical advice, and failure to attend antenatal care.

Q9: At face value, it appears that women having three or more antenatal care (ANC) visits are more likely to die than women with fewer or no ANC visits. One possible explanation for this unexpected finding is that the women who died experienced problems in pregnancy that led them to seek antenatal care. These women may have experienced more severe complications that forced them to seek care at several points during their pregnancy, thus increasing their number of ANC visits. Another possible explanation is that, out of fear of being blamed for the death, families may have reported ANC visits that did not actually take place.

Q10: The top three causes of maternal deaths in this setting are hemorrhage (58 antepartum + 178 postpartum = 236 cases, or 33%), hypertension (114 cases, or 16%), and sepsis (60 cases, or 8%).

Sixty cases of maternal deaths were associated with genital sepsis, contributing to 8% of all maternal deaths (60 ÷ 718), and 12% of direct obstetric deaths (60 ÷ 499).

The most commonly identified avoidable factor in sepsis-related deaths was substandard care from dayas, or traditional birth attendants (22 cases, or 37%). Other commonly identified avoidable factors in sepsis-related deaths were substandard care from the obstetric team (21 cases, or 35%) and delay in seeking medical care (18 cases, or 30%).

Sepsis-related deaths accounted for the largest percentage of all cause-specific maternal deaths associated with dayas (37%). Because the majority of Egyptian women are delivered by traditional birth attendants, interventions such as the implementation of daya training programs that focus on the detection, management, and prevention of specific pregnancy-related complications, the teaching of simple hygiene principles, and the provision of appropriate maternity kits could significantly reduce maternal mortality in this setting.

Q11: On the basis of the major conclusions of this study, the following recommendations may be appropriate:

- Repeat the study on a regular basis to monitor progress in improving maternal health and to increase awareness of the problem.
- Give first priority to tackling problems within hospital facilities, such as improvements in essential obstetric functions (i.e., addressing the supply side of health care).
- Develop and use protocols (i.e., posters and flowcharts) for the management of common obstetric emergencies, such as signs of nonprogressive or obstructed labor, the need for IV fluid replacement, the use of aseptic techniques, suitable antibiotic treatment, and aggressive management of acute infections.
- Further investigate the precise reasons for delay in seeking care.
- Involve senior obstetricians in obstetric care, especially in making early decisions for operative procedures.
- Perform hospital audits to identify administrative and management problems.
- Actively involve teaching hospitals of the Ministry of Health in postgraduate training and qualification programs.
- Continue and strengthen daya training programs.
- Implement campaigns to improve women's awareness of their own health.

www.ingramcontent.com/pod-product-compliance
Lightning Source LLC
Chambersburg PA
CBHW081840170526
45167CB00007B/2864